Everyday Diabetes in Primary Care

A Case-Based Approach

Everyday Diabetes in Primary Care

A Case-Based Approach

Jay H. Shubrook, DO, FACOFP, FAAFP

Professor, Primary Care Department
Diabetologist
Touro University California
College of Osteopathic Medicine
Vallejo, California

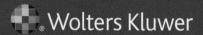 Wolters Kluwer

Philadelphia • Baltimore • New York • London
Buenos Aires • Hong Kong • Sydney • Tokyo

Senior Acquisitions Editor: Joe Cho
Development Editor: Maria M. McAvey
Editorial Coordinator: Anju Radhakrishnan
Marketing Manager: Kirsten Watrud
Production Project Manager: Matt West
Design Manager: Stephen Druding
Manufacturing Coordinator: Lisa Bowling
Prepress Vendor: TNQ Technologies

9 8 7 6 5 4 3 2 1

Printed in Mexico.

Library of Congress Cataloging-in-Publication Data

ISBN-13: 978-1-975209-84-1

Cataloging in Publication data available on request from publisher.

shop.lww.com

This is dedicated to Sam, Jessie, and Casey. You are my greatest inspiration. Thank you for believing in me.

Foreword

I have spent many years as part of various national and international writing groups for diagnosing and treating people with diabetes, of all sorts. Part of the reason I join these committees is to learn from the experts and be privy to the considerations that go into deciding what is best. Recently I was part of the ADA/EASD Writing Group for the Management of Type 1 Diabetes in Adults. The topic I was most interested in was how to diagnose type 1 diabetes in an adult. I was sure there was something I was missing. When I was a medical student, type 1 diabetes was easier to diagnose. It happened in children who were lean, who presented in diabetic ketoacidosis (DKA) and ended up on insulin for the rest of their lives because they make no endogenous insulin. But now?

Now we know that half of all type 1 diabetes is diagnosed in adults. Those adults are lean, overweight, or obese (approximately 30% in each group). Many have positive autoantibodies, but some do not. And having positive autoantibodies does not diagnose type 1 diabetes because people with type 2 diabetes can also have positive autoantibodies. Some people with type 1 diabetes present with DKA but most do not. And of those who present with DKA, some have type 2 diabetes. In people under the age of 35 what we think is type 1 diabetes can actually be maturity-onset diabetes of the young (MODY); however, all our data on the genetics of MODY and type 1 diabetes come from studies in non-Hispanic white individuals living in Northern Europe, particularly the United Kingdom. We have no idea what rates are in Hispanic white, black, or Asian populations. Finally, we used to think that after 5 years of having type 1 diabetes C-peptide levels would be very low or unmeasurable and now we know that in 25% of people who have had type 1 diabetes for 40 years or more still have measurable C-peptide levels.

I have heard that we are seeing many more adults with autoantibody-negative new-onset type 1 diabetes than ever before. So what is a clinician to do? Trust their clinical judgment and learn from what others do. And the best way to learn is from others who see many many people with diabetes, because there is no one correct way to diagnose many the increasingly different subtypes of diabetes that present themselves in our patients. In my practice I see more "atypical" forms of diabetes than typical ones and with the increase in validated genetic testing we may well find thousands of different subtypes of both type 1 and type 2 diabetes.

In this book, Dr. Shubrook draws on his experience and shares many cases to teach readers how to approach each patient and their unique needs. As always, the key is to do no harm. To keep people safe and avoid DKA, use insulin. But don't be afraid to safely titrate it up and down, try other agents, and learn from how the patient responds to therapy. What works in one phase of a person's life may not work in another. And don't be afraid to ask a colleague for an opinion. Finally, teach your patients to be their own advocates, to ask questions but to always be clear on what their treatment goals are because maintaining health is a lifelong endeavor, not something that should ever be ignored. This book should help you manage your patients more individually and effectively and learn from Dr. Shubrook, one of the leading diabetes clinicians of our times.

Anne Peters, MD
Professor of Clinical Medicine
Director of the USC Clinical Diabetes Programs
Keck School of Medicine of the University of Southern California

Preface

Diabetes has become a noncommunicable pandemic. No matter where a health care professional practices medicine today, they will need to treat people with diabetes. This book is intended for the busy primary care clinician, to help inform their day-to-day management of patients with diabetes. This text will also be a useful resource for diabetes educators, dietitians, clinical pharmacists, and medical residents, and relevant to anyone involved in the treatment and/or prevention of diabetes, including engaged active patients and family members. Some important topics covered in this book include utilizing the initial presentation to determine the specific type of diabetes, optimizing patient-centered care to help engage in initial care and long-term diabetes self-management, and highlighting best practices in the use of diabetes medications and technologies. I hope you find this immediately useful in your practice.

Acknowledgments

My sincere gratitude to Robert Gotfried, DO, Elizabeth Beverly, PhD, and Samantha Shubrook, MA, for their heavy editing of this book. Their editing helped to keep the material interesting, accurate, and inclusive.

Contents

Introduction

While most people think only of type 1 and type 2 diabetes, there are actually many forms of diabetes. Diabetes types are generally unified by hyperglycemia, but their pathogenesis can be quite distinct. Because primary care clinicians provide the overwhelming majority of diabetes care, it is essential that they know how to identify and treat the various forms. This first chapter examines the value of clinical presentations. When the clinician is aware of the different forms of diabetes, they are better able to identify key features and make correct diagnoses.

Case 1. Type 2 Diabetes in Adults

"My heart attack gave me diabetes."

A 58-year-old man recently presented to the emergency room with substernal chest pain that began while he was working in the yard. The chest pain was associated with nausea, diaphoresis, and shortness of breath. He had an anterior wall STEMI (ST-elevation myocardial infarction). This was successfully treated with PTCA (percutaneous transluminal coronary angioplasty)/stent placement. While he was in the hospital, he was surprised to learn that he had diabetes. This was not part of his medical history in the past. His glucose in the emergency room was 234 mg/dL and his hemoglobin A1c was 8.4%. Glucose readings in the hospital ran between 150 and 260 mg/dL. He presented 1 week later for hospital follow-up.

Prior to the hospitalization he had no known past medical history and was not taking any medications regularly. In the hospital, he was put on a statin, angiotensin-converting enzyme inhibitor (ACEI), and an antiplatelet agent.

Medications (prescribed on discharge): metformin 500 mg bid (not started this yet), lipitor 40 mg daily, clopidogrel 75 mg daily, lisinopril 20 mg daily, and ASA (acetylsalicylic acid) 325 mg daily

Allergies: none

Family Medical History: premature atherosclerotic cardiovascular disease, hypertension, dyslipidemia, and type 2 diabetes in his family; his brother and his father both had myocardial infarctions in their 50s.

Social History: nonsmoker, drinks 2 to 4 beers 3 times per week after work, fast-food diet priorly, no regular physical activity, lives with his wife of 25 years; he works as an accountant.

He wants to understand if he really does have diabetes. He has heard that statins give people diabetes and is wondering if this happened to him. Since coming home, his wife has put him on a very strict low-fat, calorie-controlled diet. He is scheduled to start cardiac rehab next week. He was given a glucometer upon discharge but not shown how to use it, so he has not started checking his blood sugars at home.

Physical Exam: Ht. 5′7″, Wt. 195 lb, BMI 30.5, T 98.6, P 88, R 15, BP 125/80

CV: heart rate and rhythm are regular; normal peripheral pulses, no bruits

RESP: lungs CTA anterior and posterior

Skin: bruising noted in left groin from his cardiac catheterization

Otherwise: normal exam

Lab Values (from hospital):

Comprehensive Metabolic Panel	Value	Reference Range
Sodium	141	136-145 mmol/L
Potassium, serum	4.2	3.5-5.3 mmol/L
Chloride, serum	99	98-110 mmol/L
Carbon dioxide (CO_2)	26	19-30 mmol/L
Urea nitrogen, blood (BUN)	15	7-25 mg/dL
Creatinine, serum	0.64	0.5-1.10 mg/dL
Estimated glomerular filtration rate (eGFR)	104	>60 mL/min/1.73 m²
Glucose, serum	225	65-99 mg/dL
Calcium, serum	9.9	8.6-10.2 mg/dL
Protein, total	7.1	6.1-8.1 g/dL
Albumin	4.3	3.6-4.1 g/dL
Globulin	2.8	1.9-3.7 g/dL
AST (SGOT)	56	10-35 U/L
ALT (SGPT)	50	6-29 U/L
Bilirubin, total	0.7	0.2-1.2 mg/dL
Alkaline phosphatase	100	33-115 U/L

Lipid Panel	Value	Reference Range
Cholesterol, total	248	125-200 mg/dL
Triglycerides	244	<150 mg/dL
LDL (calculated)	148	<130 mg/dL
HDL cholesterol	38	>40 mg/dL men; >50 women
Non-HDL cholesterol	198	<130

Other Labs	Value	Reference Range
HbA1c	8.4%	<5.7% (normal)
Urine albumin/creatinine ratio (UACr)	88 mg/G	<30 mg/g

 CASE QUESTIONS

1. Does he indeed have diabetes mellitus?
2. Is his presentation common for type 2 diabetes mellitus?
3. Did the statin give him diabetes?
4. How to tell your patient that he does in fact have type 2 diabetes?
5. What are the next steps for this patient?

ANSWERS AND EXPLANATIONS

1. While the diagnosis of diabetes usually requires two tests separated by time, the fact that he has an elevated random glucose well above 200 mg/dL and hemoglobin A1c at 8.4% confirms that he has had hyperglycemia for a minimum of 3 months prior to the lab test. Repeating any of the qualifying labs to confirm the diagnosis is an option including a fasting glucose, a 2-hour postprandial glucose, a glucose tolerance test (GTT), or a hemoglobin A1c. However, considering his current levels, this is largely unnecessary (Table 1.1 and Figure 1.1).

2. More than 10% of the US adult population had diabetes mellitus in 2020. Another 35% had prediabetes.[3] Importantly, more than 20% of those individuals with active diabetes mellitus did not know they had diabetes (undiagnosed).[4]

   The most common presentation of type 2 diabetes is an asymptomatic finding on a routine screening lab. It is also worth noting that one-third of people with diabetes find out that they have diabetes in association with the presentation of a diabetes-related complication. It has also been reported that 25% of people who present with a heart attack find out that they have diabetes at that time.[3]

3. While there have been reports that statins can raise glucose levels and even tip someone into new onset type 2 diabetes, it is very unlikely in this case. Prior to his hospitalization, he was not taking any medications and his glucose and A1c were elevated. The short period of time he took the statin in the hospital would not have had a significant impact on his glucose and HbA1c.

   A 2009 study looked at changes in glucose from statin use in people with and without diabetes. The net increase in fasting glucose was 7 mg/dL in people with known diabetes and 2 mg/dL in people without diabetes.[5,6] While this is a significant increase, the benefits from statins far outweigh the potential adverse effect of hyperglycemia. It is unlikely that statins will increase this risk in people who do not have insulin resistance already.[7] It is worth noting that this study was completed within the Veterans health system, which is known to have substantially higher rates of diabetes and prediabetes.[6]

4. Denial, fear, and anger are common reactions to being diagnosed with a serious health condition, like diabetes. If the diagnosis is unexpected, as in the case for this patient, he may try to find an alternative explanation or minimize its importance. This is a normal way of coping when first diagnosed; however, if the denial or

TABLE 1.1	Diagnostic Criteria for Diabetes[1]	
Normal	**Prediabetes**	**Diabetes**
Fasting glucose <100 mg/dL	Impaired fasting glucose ≥100-125 mg/dL	Fasting glucose ≥126 mg/dL
2-h postmeal glucose (PG) < 140 mg/dL	Impaired glucose tolerance 2-h PG ≥ 140-199 mg/dL	2-h PG ≥ 200 mg Random PG ≥ 200 + symptoms
A1c < 5.7%	5.7%-6.4%	≥6.5%

Based on American Diabetes Association. *Standards of Medical Care 2022. Classification and Diagnosis and of Diabetes.*
https://diabetesjournals.org/care/article/45/Supplement_1/S17/138925/2-Classification-and-Diagnosis-of-Diabetes

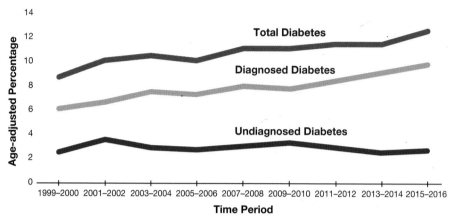

FIGURE 1.1. Trends in age-adjusted prevalence of diagnosed diabetes, undiagnosed diabetes, and total diabetes among adults aged 18 years or older, United States, 1999 to 2016. Diagnosed diabetes was based on self-report. Undiagnosed diabetes was based on fasting plasma glucose and A1c levels among people self-reporting no diabetes. (Reproduced from CDC. *Prevalence of Both Diagnosed and Undiagnosed Diabetes*. 2021. https://www.cdc.gov/diabetes/data/statistics-report/diagnosed-undiagnosed-diabetes.html.)

minimization of diabetes goes on too long, your patient will increase the likelihood of serious diabetes complications. This is particularly relevant for this case given adult men tend to have the most difficulty accepting a diagnosis of diabetes. As a clinician, the best coping strategies you can offer your patient are to go slow with recommendations for diet and physical activity modification (everything does not need to be fixed overnight), manage stress and anxiety, refer to diabetes education, identify the right support network, and involve family members in the management plan.[8]

5. His recovery should start with cardiac rehabilitation including diabetes education, medical nutrition therapy, moderation of alcohol intake, and encouragement to participate in at least 150 minutes of moderately vigorous physical activity per week.

Concomitant pharmacotherapy should also be initiated. Historically, this approach includes the use of metformin as foundational therapy, which certainly could be used in this case. However, in light of recent cardiovascular outcome trials and changes in guidelines, this patient also has a compelling indication for a medication that has been shown to have benefit to reduce secondary atherosclerotic cardiovascular events. These medications could include one of the SGLT-2 (sodium-glucose cotransporter-2) inhibitors or GLP (glucagon-like peptide)-1 receptor agonists with proven benefit in cardiovascular risk reduction.[9] We will discuss this topic much more later in the book (see Chapter 4 for further discussion on this point).

Case Summary and Closing Points

Type 2 diabetes is a common and, for many, a silent condition. Since most people have no symptoms early in the disease, it is common for clinicians to find and diagnose people at the time of a complication. This may be microvascular (retinopathy, nephropathy, neuropathy) or macrovascular (acute coronary syndrome or stroke). The key to identifying type 2 diabetes as early as possible is to know the risk factors and use the evidence-based screening recommendations.

References

1. American Diabetes Association. *Standards of Medical Care 2022. Classification and Diagnosis and of Diabetes*; 2021. https://diabetesjournals.org/care/article/45/Supplement_1/S17/138925/2-Classification-and-Diagnosis-of-Diabetes
2. CDC. *Prevalence of Both Diagnosed and Undiagnosed Diabetes*; 2021. https://www.cdc.gov/diabetes/data/statistics-report/diagnosed-undiagnosed-diabetes.html
3. Norhammar A, Tenerz A, Nilsson G, et al. Glucose metabolism in patients with acute myocardial infarction and no previous diagnosis of diabetes mellitus: a prospective study. *Lancet*. 2002;359(9324):2140-2144. doi:10.1016/S0140-6736(02)09089-X
4. CDC. Diabetes Fact Sheet. https://www.cdc.gov/diabetes/data/statistics-report/diagnosed-undiagnosed-diabetes.html
5. Sukhija R, Prayaga S, Marashdeh M, et al. Effect of statins on fasting plasma glucose in diabetic and nondiabetic patients. *J Invest Med*. 2009;57:495-499.
6. Liu Y, Sayam S, Shao X, et al. Prevalence of and Trends in diabetes among Veterans, United States, 2005-2014. *Prev Chronic Dis*. 2017;14:E135. doi:10.5888/pcd14.170230
7. Chogtu B, Magazine R, Bairy KL. Statin use and risk of diabetes mellitus. *World J Diabetes*. 2015;6(2):352-357. doi:10.4239/wjd.v6.i2.352
8. Mathew R, Gucciardi E, De Melo M, Barata P. Self-management experiences among men and women with type 2 diabetes mellitus: a qualitative analysis. *BMC Fam Pract*. 2012;13:122. doi:10.1186/1471-2296-13-122
9. American Diabetes Association. Standards of Medical Care 2022. Pharmacologic Approach to Glycemic Control. https://diabetesjournals.org/care/article/45/Supplement_1/S125/138908/9-Pharmacologic-Approaches-to-Glycemic-Treatment

Case 2. Type 2 Diabetes in Adolescents

"Where did this rash come from?"

A 14-year-old African American boy presented (with his parents) with concerns about a rash (Figure 1.2). The rash was present on his posterior neck. They were not sure how long it had been there. Recently, his teacher called with concerns about hygiene. He has a history of allergic rhinitis and takes loratadine 10 mg daily as needed.

He was born at term and weighed 9 lb 4 oz. (4196 g). He met all his normal developmental milestones. He has been "big" for as long as the family can remember, noting that his weight gain accelerated starting at age 12.

Medications: loratadine

Allergies: none (medication, latex, food)

Family Medical History: type 2 diabetes in mom, maternal grandmother (MGM), and paternal grandmother (PGM); asthma in dad and brother

Social History: Lives at home with parents and younger sister. Currently in ninth grade. Doing "only ok" at school. Has socially withdrawn this year. No tobacco, alcohol, or recreational drugs. He eats school-supported breakfast and lunch (mom reports this is not usually healthy—pizza, sloppy joes, fries—but they need the help). No regular physical activity. He enjoys online video games. The family's goal for today's visit is to "get rid of this rash."

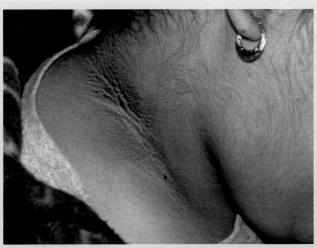

FIGURE 1.2. Picture of skin lesions. (Used with permission from Goodheart H. *Goodheart's Same-Site Differential Diagnosis*, 2nd ed. 2022. Wolters Kluwer.)

Physical Exam: Ht. 5′6″, Wt. 293 lb, BMI 47.3, T 98.6, P 88, R 15, BP 138/80

CV/RESP: exam normal

Skin: velvety hyperpigmented plaques along posterior neck and axilla; pink striae noted on the abdomen and shoulders

GEN: pleasant but withdrawn male; truncal obesity

Prediabetes/Diabetes Diagnosis:

Normal	Prediabetes	Diabetes
Fasting glucose < 100 mg/dL	Impaired fasting glucose ≥ 100-125 mg/dL	Fasting glucose ≥ 126 mg/dL
2-h postmeal glucose (PG) < 140 mg/dL	Impaired glucose tolerance 2-h PG ≥ 140-199 mg/dL	2-h PG ≥200 mg Random PG ≥ 200 + symptoms
A1C < 5.7%	5.7%-6.4%	≥6.5%

Adapted from the ADA SOC Diagnostic Criteria for Diabetes: American Diabetes Association. *Standards of Medical Care 2022. Classification and Diagnosis and of Diabetes.* https://diabetesjournals.org/care/article/45/Supplement_1/S17/138925/2-Classification-and-Diagnosis-of-Diabetes

Ⓠ CASE QUESTIONS

1. What is the problem list for this patient?
2. Does he have diabetes? If so, what type?
3. What is causing the rash?
4. What are the next steps?

ANSWERS AND EXPLANATIONS

1. The problem list for this patient includes:
   a. Obesity
   b. Metabolic syndrome
   c. Type 2 diabetes
   d. Suspected nonalcoholic fatty liver disease
   e. Albuminuria
   f. Concern about depression

2. His glucose value and hemoglobin A1c clearly indicate that he has diabetes. Given that he has a family history of type 2 diabetes, his body habitus matches type 2 diabetes. Further, the fact that he has dyslipidemia and presents with physical characteristics of insulin resistance, the overwhelming likelihood is that he has type 2 diabetes. While it is often thought that children only get type 1 diabetes, we now know that a sizable proportion of children diagnosed with diabetes actually have type 2 diabetes.[1] Pediatric obesity is becoming an increasingly common scenario and a significant public health challenge. We are seeing more and more obese adolescents and young adults being diagnosed with metabolic-related diseases such as type 2 diabetes.[1,2]

   Given the clinical presentation, there is no need to do any additional evaluation at this time. If he were to develop catabolic symptoms later, he could be tested for type 1 diabetes (Figure 1.3).

3. The skin changes are from acanthosis nigricans, a problem related to insulin resistance. It is most commonly seen on the neck, especially the posterior aspect of the neck in the axilla and sometimes in the groin. It may also occur on extensor surfaces.[3]

   The pathophysiology of acanthosis is believed to be related to the excessive stimulation of epidermal keratinocytes and dermal fibroblasts. This stimulation is felt to be a result of excess endogenous insulin and insulin-like growth factor.[4] These hormones rise with obesity and insulin resistance. Insulin is itself a growth factor, and it stimulates growth of many cell lines including melanin cells in the epidermis. The skin changes of plaque formation and hyperpigmentation appear when the growth rate exceeds the sloughing of cells causing the skin to thicken and becomes darker.

   This rash is often mistaken for dirt or poor hygiene. It is important to recognize that there is no specific agreed upon treatment for acanthosis other than interventions that improve insulin resistance.

4. There is much to consider here. It is important to explain to the patient and his family that acanthosis is a marker of high genetic risk for insulin resistance and type 2 diabetes. This helps to direct attention away from issues about weight and focus on the genetic component of type 2 diabetes. It is important to reinforce that the rash is not hygiene related. It is also important to communicate that there are no simple or direct solutions for the skin changes. The best approach is to address the underlying cause and provide accurate medical information and psychosocial support. Diabetes care guidelines recommended screening adolescents for depression at diagnosis and routine follow-up. Adolescents with type 2 diabetes are at higher risk for depression compared to the general adolescent population. Your patient

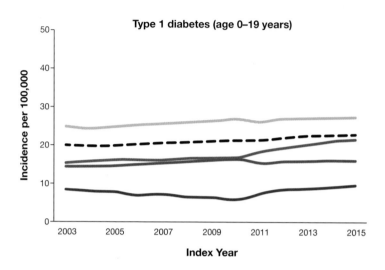

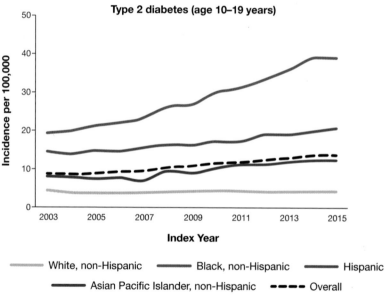

FIGURE 1.3. Trends in the incidence of type 1 and type 2 diabetes in youth, overall and by race/ethnicity, 2002 to 2015. (Adapted Divers J, Mayer-Davis EJ, Lawrence JM, et al. Trends in incidence of type 1 and type 2 diabetes among youths—selected counties and Indian reservations, United States, 2002-2015. *MMWR Morb Mortal Wkly Rep.* 2020;69(6):161-165. doi:10.15585/mmwr.mm6906a3)

indicates that he has been more socially withdrawn this year in school, which suggests potential psychosocial concerns. Screening and diagnosing depression is critical given symptoms of depression interfere with the ability to engage in self-care behaviors, like physical activity, following a healthy diet, managing weight, and monitoring blood glucose levels.

This adolescent and family need a family-based comprehensive approach to address the items noted above with a particular focus on mental health and healthy coping. (This approach will be explored in Chapter 2, Case 2.)

Case Summary and Closing Points

This is a case wherein the initial presentation of type 2 diabetes is not glucose-related. It is worth remembering that skin changes are commonly the first signs of diabetes especially in at-risk populations. Further, it is important to remember that when type 2 diabetes is diagnosed in adolescents and young adults the condition is more severe and should be treated promptly and thoroughly. Optimally, this includes a team-based approach that addresses the health needs of the entire family.

References

1. Mayer-Davis EJ, Lawrence JM, Dabelea D, et al. Incidence Trends of type 1 and type 2 diabetes among youths, 2002-2012. *N Engl J Med.* 2017;376(15):1419-1429.
2. Divers J, Mayer-Davis EJ, Lawrence JM, et al. Trends in incidence of type 1 and type 2 diabetes among youths—selected counties and Indian reservations, United States, 2002-2015. *MMWR Morb Mortal Wkly Rep.* 2020;69(6):161-165. doi:10.15585/mmwr.mm6906a3
3. Duff M, Demidova O, Blackburn S, Shubrook JH. Cutaneous manifestations of diabetes. *Clin Diabetes.* 2015;33(1):40-48.
4. Hines A, Alavi A, Davis MDP. Cutaneous manifestations of diabetes. *Med Clin North Am.* 2021;105(4):681-697. doi:10.1016/j.mcna.2021.04.008
5. Anderson BJ, McKay SV. Psychosocial issues in youth with type 2 diabetes mellitus. *Curr Diab Rep.* 2009;9:147-153.

Case 3.   Type 1 Diabetes in Children

"We thought he had the flu."

An 8-year-old boy presented to the emergency room with a stomach flu that did not seem to be resolving. His mom explained that he started acting differently a couple of weeks ago. He came home from a sleepover, and she noticed that he was drinking a lot and peeing a lot. He also seemed to be more hungry than normal. These behaviors persisted for several weeks. Also, mom noticed that he was losing weight. While changes in eating were common for him with growth spurts, weight loss was not. More recently things worsened, as he complained of abdominal pain and nausea and vomited several times.

Medications: none

Allergies: none

Family Medical History: immediate family in good health; Alzheimer disease in MGM

Social History: lives with his parents, one older sister, and one younger brother; normal developmental milestones; picky eater; doing well in school, fourth grade.

Physical Exam: in emergency room

Vitals: HR 124, R 28, T 98.6 F, BP 90/60, Ht. 52 in, Wt. 54 lb, BMI 16

General: appears dehydrated, lying on gurney, sluggish but cooperative

HEENT: oral mucosa dry and breath smells "fruity"; eyes appear sunken

CV: rapid but regular

RESP: clear with Kussmaul breathing

Abdomen: BS (bowel sounds) active, mild diffuse tenderness, no localization

Neuro: he is arousable, oriented to person and place; no focal neurologic deficits or nuchal rigidity

Lab Values:

CBC	Value	Reference Range
White blood cell count	18	3.8-10.8 thousand/µL
Red blood cell count	4.8	3.8-5.10 million/µL
Hemoglobin	14.3	12.6-17 g/dL
Hematocrit	48%	37%-51%
MCV (mean corpuscular volume)	91	80-100 fL
MCH (mean corpuscular hemoglobin)	29.9	27-33 pg
MCHC (mean corpuscular hemoglobin concentration)	32.9	32-36 g/dL
RDW (red cell distribution width)	12.7	1%-15%
Platelet count	336	140-400 thousand/µL
Absolute neutrophils	9000	1500-7800 cells/µL
Absolute lymphocytes	1600	850-3900
Absolute monocytes	375	200-950
Absolute eosinophils	75	15-500
Absolute basophils	43	0-200
Neutrophils	90	%
Lymphocytes	10	%
Monocytes	3	%
Eosinophils	2	%
Basophils	1	%
Bands	4	0%-10%

Comprehensive Metabolic Panel	Value	Reference Range
Glucose	450	70-99 mg/dL
Blood urea nitrogen (BUN)	44	7-25 mg/dL
Creatinine	2.0	0.5-1.10 mg/dL
eGFR-est	56	>60 mL/min/1.73 m^2
Sodium	140	136-145 mEq/L

Comprehensive Metabolic Panel	Value	Reference Range
Potassium	5.0	3.5-5.3 mEq/L
Chloride	98	98-110 mEq/L
Bicarbonate	10	19-30 mEq/L
Anion gap	32	7-13 mEq/L
Calcium	10.3	8.6-10.3 mg/dL
Protein total	7.1	6-8.3 g/dL
Albumin	4.0	3.6-5.1 g/dL
Bilirubin total	1.0	0.2-1.2 mg/dL
AST	15	10-35 IU/L
ALT	12	9-46 IU/L
Alkaline phosphatase	45	40-115 IU/L
Lipase	20	0-160 U
Magnesium	1.9	1.7-2.2 mg/dL
Phosphorus	2	2.5-4.5 mg/dL
Beta hydroxyl butyrate	3.5	<0.5 mmol/L
Lactic acid	1	0.5-1 mmol/L
Serum osmolality	321	285-295 mmol/kg H_2O
Alcohol level	negative	<10 mg/dL
Salicylate level	negative	2-10 mg/dL
Hemoglobin A1c	9.6%	<5.7%
		5.7%-6.4%—increased risk for diabetes

Arterial Blood Gas	Value	Reference Range
pH	6.9	7.35-7.45
pCO_2	23	35-45 mm Hg
pO_2	80	75-100 mm Hg
HCO_3^-	10	22 -28 mEq/L
O_2 saturation	95	94%-100%

Urine Analysis	Value	Reference Range
Color	Straw	
Appearance	Clear	
pH	4	4.6-8
Specific gravity	>1.030	1.005-1.030
Glucose	800 mg/dL	Negative
Ketones	Large	None to small
Blood	Negative	

Urine Analysis	Value	Reference Range
Bilirubin	Negative	
Urobilinogen	Negative	
Nitrite	Negative	
Leukocyte esterase	Negative	
Rapid COVID-19 Test	Negative	
Rapid influenza screen	Negative	
Urine drug screen	Negative	
Blood cultures	Report pending	

 CASE QUESTIONS

1. What is making him sick?
2. Does he have diabetes? If so, what type?
3. What are best practices for communicating with the family regarding a new diagnosis of diabetes?
4. What are the next steps?

 ANSWERS AND EXPLANATIONS

1. This child has the "polys," a presentation of polyuria, polydipsia, and polyphagia with weight loss. This is the classic presentation of type 1 diabetes. According to clinical presentation and labs, he is in an anion gap ketoacidosis—mostly likely diabetic ketoacidosis (DKA).

   When severe hyperglycemia arises from an absolute deficiency of insulin, the body starts to use alternate fuels such as ketones to fuel the brain and other key areas. This process causes unopposed lipolysis and oxidation of free fatty acids and thereby results in ketone body production and a subsequent increased anion gap metabolic acidosis. If insulin deficiency is persistent and hyperglycemia becomes prominent, the body starts to develop catabolic symptoms (the "polys") and weight loss. If this persists, the body becomes acidotic. Acidosis can commonly lead to symptoms such as nausea, abdominal pain, and vomiting. Most people who present with DKA as their initial finding of diabetes assume that something else is causing these symptoms such as a stomach flu.

   Once the acidosis is treated, his gastrointestinal symptoms are likely to get better. He also needs fluid resuscitation. Once the fluid deficit is treated and he receives an adequate amount of insulin to prevent catabolic symptoms, his "polys" will improve.

2. Glucose screening for diabetes when a child is sick is not optimal as children can have substantial hyperglycemia under severe stress.[1] In this case, with a concomitant HbA1c of 9.6%, we know that the patient has been hyperglycemic for 3 months—even longer than his poly symptoms. We can confidently diagnose him with diabetes based on this and his presentation in DKA.

   DKA is one of the most common presentations of new diagnosis of type 1 diabetes. Based on his lack of family history of diabetes and the presentation at age 8 with DKA, with no signs of insulin resistance, he likely has type 1 diabetes. However, there are a couple of factors to keep in mind. There is a ketosis-prone (DKA-prone) form of type 2 diabetes, albeit this is more common in young adults who are phenotypically more like type 2. Further, COVID-19 infections have been shown to increase rates of type 1 and type 2 diabetes as well as cases of sustained hyperglycemia that eventually completely resolve.[2,3]

His presentation is most consistent with type 1 diabetes. He should be treated as having type 1 diabetes in both the inpatient and outpatient setting until further evaluation can be completed when he is more stable.

3. Receiving a lifelong diagnosis like type 1 diabetes can be a traumatic experience for the family as well as the child. The most important thing to communicate while the child is in DKA is the child appears to have type 1 diabetes; the most immediate concern is to stabilize them; and there will be an opportunity to discuss their condition and its implications once the child is stabilized—typically the next day. Providing more information on the first day is not likely to be beneficial, as the shock of the diagnosis and the child's condition fully occupies the family's attention. Waiting to start diabetes education when the child is more stable is important as it allows all relevant family members to be present, improves their ability to hear the messaging, and allows everyone in the family to take in the same information. This is especially important as there are many misconceptions about what causes type 1 diabetes and what constitutes optimal treatment.

Important messages on day 2 (when the family can be assembled with the child and the child is feeling better) include the following: (1) the type of diabetes (if known); (2) how it will be treated; (3) information about whether or not it can be cured; and (4) the specific and likely impacts on the child's and family's daily activities. Related to message 4, the child and his family may experience a variety of feelings—fear, anger, guilt, helplessness, anxiety, etc.—about the diagnosis and what's to come. As a provider, you can help the child and family cope with the diagnosis by acknowledging their feelings and reinforcing that the child will continue to be a contributing member of society.

Common education and treatment goals before discharge include (1) the ability of the child and key family members to check glucose, inject insulin, and check ketones; (2) knowledge of common symptoms of hyperglycemia and hypoglycemia; and (3) knowledge of how to treat hyperglycemia and hypoglycemia. There is much more to learn, but these basics are most critical to help the family feel safe enough to go home.

4. Both the child and their family will have to learn many new skills and incorporate them into their daily lives for the rest of the child's life. Recognizing the enormity of this situation, it is essential to practice patience while providing instruction for small steps that the family can achieve in a timely manner. These new skills include learning about carbohydrates, glucose monitoring, and calculating and injecting insulin—this will include basal insulin, mealtime insulin, and correction insulin. The child and family members will need to learn how to identify and treat hyperglycemia and hypoglycemia (as stated above).

All of the organizations that interact with the child will also need written instructions on how to assist the child (school, day care, extracurricular activities).

A newly diagnosed child can expect to be seen every 3 to 5 days for the first 2 weeks. Children and family members should be encouraged to bring in questions with the goal of honing their abilities incrementally. Early diabetes education, in the hospital and at home, is critically important to build a strong set of diabetes self-care skills increasing the comfort and confidence of the child and family.

Case Summary and Closing Points

Receiving a diagnosis of type 1 diabetes is often a traumatic experience for the person being diagnosed and the family involved. The most important thing health care professionals can do to help the family is to provide accurate information and a comprehensive treatment plan including diabetes education and nutrition education. The focus of care should be helping the person live life as normally as possible with their diabetes rather than allowing their diabetes to dictate what they do and when.

References

1. Srinivasan V. Stress hyperglycemia in pediatric critical illness: the intensive care unit adds to the stress! *J Diabetes Sci Technol.* 2012;6(1):37-47. doi:10.1177/193229681200600106
2. Khunti K, Del Prato S, Mathieu C, Kahn SE, Gabbay RA, Buse JB. COVID-19, hyperglycemia, and new-onset diabetes. *Diabetes Care.* 2021;44(12):2645-2655. doi:10.2337/dc21-1318
3. Cromer SJ, Colling C, Schatoff D, et al. Newly diagnosed diabetes vs. pre-existing diabetes upon admission for COVID-19: associated factors, short-term outcomes, and long-term glycemic phenotypes. *J Diabetes Complications.* 2022;36(4):108145. ISSN 1056-8727. doi:10.1016/j.jdiacomp.2022.108145

Case 4. Latent Autoimmune Diabetes in Adults (LADA) Clinical Presentation

"I just cannot eat any carbs."

A 48-year-old woman presented to discuss her diabetes treatment. She explained that she had a past medical history of hypothyroidism and anemia. She was diagnosed with hypothyroidism at age 40 years when she was losing her hair and experiencing fatigue. She takes levothyroxine 75 μg daily for hypothyroidism.

She reported that she was diagnosed with diabetes after routine lab testing to monitor her hypothyroidism. Her physician started her on metformin, but, despite trying multiple formulations and doses, she had to stop as she could not tolerate the gastrointestinal side effects. She is currently taking glimepiride 4 mg daily and pioglitazone 30 mg daily each morning. She tried taking higher doses of glimepiride, but she had too many hypoglycemic episodes.

She worked at a gas station/convenience store. As the manager, she worked long hours. She did not get much physical activity outside of work. She admitted to eating more meals at the store than she should. She felt guilty because when she saw that when she ate carbs it made her glucose skyrocket. She explained that if she ate "low carb," she could keep her glucose below 250 mg/dL. Her sleep schedule was unpredictable as a result of a fluctuating work schedule.

Medications: glimepiride 4 mg daily, pioglitazone 30 mg daily, levothyroxine 75 μg daily

Allergies: none

Family Medical History: hypothyroidism in sister and mom; no family history of diabetes

Social History: smokes 1 ppd (30 pk/y history), drinks 1× a month, and no recreational drug use; she eats a fast-food diet, reports no regular physical activity, and lives alone.

She did not check her glucose frequently—a few times a week. She had readings in the 140s to 160s when she woke up. She reported that these readings were better later in the day if she did not eat carbs, but they were higher (>200 mg/dL) if she did. She had not had any recent hypoglycemic episodes but reported that she used to get them if she drank alcohol.

Her goal for her visit was to find a treatment that would allow her to eat more normally.

Physical Exam: Ht. 5′5″, Wt. 129 lb, BMI 21.5, T 98.6, P 88, R 15, BP 110/66

HEENT: normal thyroid exam

CV: normal

RESP: normal

Skin: vitiligo noted on neck and arms

Otherwise: normal exam

Lab Values (fasting-drawn before visit):

Comprehensive Metabolic Panel	Value	Reference Range
Sodium	141	136-145 mmol/L
Potassium, serum	4.2	3.5-5.3 mmol/L
Chloride, serum	103	98-110 mmol/L
Carbon dioxide (CO_2)	28	19-30 mmol/L
Urea nitrogen, blood (BUN)	12	7-25 mg/dL
Creatinine, serum	0.6	0.5-1.10 mg/dL
eGFR	124	>60 mL/min/1.73 m²
Glucose, serum	168	65-99 mg/dL
Calcium, serum	9.9	8.6-10.2 mg/dL
Protein, total	7.1	6.1-8.1 g/dL
Albumin	4.3	3.6-4.1 g/dL
Globulin	2.8	1.9-3.7 g/dL
AST (SGOT)	23	10-35 U/L
ALT (SGPT)	37	6-29 U/L
Bilirubin, total	0.7	0.2-1.2 mg/dL
Alkaline phosphatase	100	33-115 U/L

Lipid Panel	Value	Reference Range
Cholesterol, total	190	125-200 mg/dL
Triglycerides	145	<150 mg/dL
LDL (calculated)	120	<130 mg/dL
HDL cholesterol	55	>40 mg/dL men; >50 women
Non-HDL cholesterol	135	<130

Other Labs	Value	Reference Range
HbA1c	8.8%	<5.7% (normal)
TSH/free T4	0.98/1.42	0.4-4.5 mIU/L/0.8-1.8 µg/dL
Urine albumin/creatinine ratio (UACr)	376 mg/G	<30 mg/G

 CASE QUESTIONS

1. What type of diabetes does she have?
2. What clinical findings (history and physical) support the diagnosis?
3. What clinical findings (lab findings) support the diagnosis?
4. What further evaluation should be completed?
5. What are the next steps?

 ANSWERS AND EXPLANATIONS

1. It is very likely that this person has a form of type 1 diabetes. Based on the history and physical, the suspicion is that she has latent autoimmune diabetes of the adult (LADA).
2. While this person was diagnosed in adulthood, she does not have the phenotype that would be consistent with type 2 diabetes, and she does not have the typical family history that would be expected. Further, she has a family history of autoimmune conditions, which would make an autoimmune condition more likely. Most people with type 2 diabetes have a family history of type 2 diabetes. Conversely, 93% of people with type 1 diabetes have no family history of diabetes.[1]

   Her physical exam is largely normal including a normal BMI, no truncal obesity, and no evidence of insulin resistance. She does have vitiligo and her thyroid exam was normal. The thyroid exam can be widely variable in patients with Hashimoto thyroiditis.
3. The great majority of people with type 2 diabetes have diabetes-related dyslipidemia, which is characterized by low HDL (high-density lipoprotein) cholesterol and high triglycerides. While it is not central to the diagnosis, many people also have high total cholesterol and LDL (low-density lipoprotein). This patient had normal lipid findings. In fact, she had a high HDL which is very unusual for someone with type 2 diabetes.
4. To confirm that she has a form of type 1 diabetes, it is prudent to measure how much insulin she makes and whether she has any markers of autoimmunity consistent with type 1 diabetes. Measures of insulin production are best completed by ordering a C-peptide in conjunction with a fasting glucose. These tests should be ordered together as the C-peptide will be responsive to the current glucose level. A high glucose level but low or undetectable C-peptide supports the conclusion of insulin deficiency.

It is also prudent to measure evidence or markers of autoimmunity consistent with type 1 diabetes. This is usually done through an autoantibody panel that includes glutamic acid decarboxylase antibodies (anti-GAD-65), insulin autoantibodies, and zinc transporter 8 antibodies. If this patient has a low C-peptide despite a high glucose and the presence of two or more autoantibodies, the likelihood of type 1 diabetes is 70% over the next 10 years and near 100% over the person's lifetime.[2]

Using the following five key features, it is possible to distinguish between an adult with type 2 diabetes and an adult with LADA:

- Age Dx less than 50 years
- Classic poly symptoms (polyuria, polydipsia, polyphagia)
- BMI < 25
- Personal history of autoimmunity
- Family history of autoimmunity

If a person meets more than two of the above criteria, then the likelihood is quite strong that they have LADA with a 90% sensitivity and a 71% specificity.[3] If they have only one or none of those features, then there is overwhelming evidence that they do not have type 1 diabetes with a 99% negative predictive value for LADA.[3]

5. Since this person has type 1 diabetes, the treatment is insulin. Currently, there is not enough evidence to support the use of oral agents for people with LADA. There are some research studies supporting the use of GLP-1 receptor agonists and pioglitazone in preserving beta cell function.[4] The clinical significance of these findings is unclear. The use of a sulfonylurea would not be beneficial for this person because it would challenge the pancreatic beta cells that are already under autoimmune attack. Therefore, insulin is the current recommended treatment for patients with LADA.

Additional Labs:

Labs	Value	Reference Range
C-peptide	0.4	0.78-1.89 ng/mL (fasting)
Islet cell antibody screen	Negative	Negative
GAD antibodies	62	<5 IU/mL
Insulin autoantibodies	<0.4	<0.4 U/mL

Case Summary and Closing Points

An asymptomatic presentation is very common with type 2 diabetes. Still, there are several key factors, as revealed in this person's history, that clinicians can be watchful for, especially in the physical exam and lab work. This patient did not have the classic type 2 diabetes phenotype or family history that would be consistent with type 2 diabetes. However, she did have a personal and family history of autoimmune disease. Her labs revealed that she did not have diabetes-related dyslipidemia. Finally, upon further evaluation, she was seen to have insulin deficiency and measures of autoimmunity, both of which confirmed the final diagnosis of a form of type 1 diabetes aka LADA (Table 1.2).

TABLE 1.2   Comparing LADA to Type 1 and Type 2 Diabetes

	T1DM	LADA	T2DM
Age of diagnosis	0-25	35-50	12 – adulthood
Time to insulin	Immediate	>6 mo	Typically years
Auto antibodies	+++	++	None
Risk for autoimmune Dx	++	+++	No added risk
Sensitivity to insulin	+++	+++	Not sensitive
Lipids	Normal	Normal	High trigs Low HDL
CV complications risk	Baseline	Elevated	Very elevated

References

1. Karges B, Prinz N, Placzek K, et al. A comparison of familial and sporadic type 1 diabetes among young patients. *Diabetes Care*. 2021;44(5):1116-1124. doi:10.2337/dc20-1829
2. Insel RA, Dunne JL, Atkinson MA, et al. Staging presymptomatic type 1 diabetes: a scientific statement of JDRF, the Endocrine Society, and the American Diabetes Association. *Diabetes Care*. 2015;38(10):1964-1974. doi:10.2337/dc15-1419
3. Fourlanos S, Perry C, Stein MS, Stankovich J, Harrison LC, Colman PG. A clinical screening tool identifies autoimmune diabetes in adults. *Diabetes Care*. 2006;29(5):970-975.
4. DeFronzo RA, Abdul-Ghani MA. Preservation of β-cell function: the key to diabetes prevention. *J Clin Endocrinol Metab*. 2011;96(8):2354-2366. doi:10.1210/jc.2011-0246

Case 5. Monogenic Diabetes

"All the women in my family get diabetes."

A 23-year-old woman presented for a refill on her medication. A year prior, she found out that she had diabetes from a work screening. At the time of her diagnosis, she felt fine and denied any "poly" symptoms or weight loss. She was not surprised by the diagnosis, though, as her sister, her mom, and MGM all were diagnosed with diabetes at a young age. Her MGM and mom both were treated with insulin. Her sister, she reported, was not very good about sticking to a treatment plan and went weeks at a time without taking insulin. This surprised her as she thought insulin was required for her diabetes type. She thinks she has type 1 but no one has ever confirmed this for her.

Medications: insulin glargine 12 units/d

Allergies: none

Family Medical History: see above; no family history of autoimmunity

Social History: no tobacco, no alcohol or recreational drugs, no over-the-counter (OTC) supplements; works as a paralegal; walks 45 to 60 minutes daily and does resistance training 2 times per week

Physical Exam: Ht. 5'5", Wt. 129 lb, BMI 21.5, T 98.6, P 80, R 18, BP 112/72

CV: heart rate and rhythm were normal

RESP: clear to auscultation

Otherwise: normal exam; no signs of insulin resistance

 CASE QUESTIONS

1. What type of diabetes does she have?
2. What clinical findings (history and physical) support the diagnosis?
3. What clinical findings (lab findings) should be ordered to support the diagnosis?
4. What are the next steps?

 ANSWERS AND EXPLANATIONS

1. She is a thin young adult. Type 1 diabetes would be a practical first guess, since she is not overweight and apparently does not require much insulin. However, she does not present with insulin deficiency with the polys. What is most unusual in this case is that many of her close relatives have diabetes. While a family history of type 2 diabetes can be expected with those with type 2, it is not common in type 1 diabetes. Further, the people in her family are thin. Her sister apparently does not take insulin regularly, yet it is well known that those with type 1 diabetes and insulin deficiency get sick quickly if they do not take insulin.

   Since she does not seem to have insulin resistance, and does not appear to have insulin deficiency, she likely has an atypical form of diabetes. Given her family history, it is most likely that she has a form of monogenic diabetes.

2. She is a young person with a strong family history, no signs of insulin resistance, and no signs of insulin deficiency.

   This is a scenario wherein ordering lab tests may be helpful to make sure she does not have type 1 (Table 1.3).

3. She makes a normal amount of insulin. She has no markers of autoimmunity, and she has a normal lipid panel.

   With this information, we need to look for other forms of diabetes since she does not appear to have autoimmunity nor insulin resistance. With her family history there is a strong likelihood of monogenic diabetes. Monogenic diabetes is present in about 1% of all people with diabetes. It is so rare that initial correct diagnosis is only made in about 6% of patients[1] (Table 1.4).

4. The first and most important step is to make sure that the patient is made aware of the type of diabetes she has and its relationship to her offspring. Since this is an autosomal dominant condition, each of her children has a 50% chance of developing this type of diabetes. Genetic testing is often needed to make a specific diagnosis and referral to a specialty center is prudent (Figure 1.4).

   Next, she has several treatment options that do not include insulin. Choosing the best treatment option often takes some time and education. This patient, for example, is facing a major change in her diagnosis and treatment paradigm. The

TABLE 1.3　Lab Values

Lipid Panel	Value	Reference Range
Cholesterol, total	188	125-200 mg/dL
Triglycerides	60	<150 mg/dL
LDL (calculated)	92	<130 mg/dL
HDL cholesterol	64	>40 mg/dL men; >50 women
Non-HDL cholesterol	108	<130

Additional Labs	Value	Reference Range
C-peptide	1.3	0.78-1.89 ng/mL (fasting)
Islet cell antibody screen	Negative	Negative
GAD antibodies	<5	<5 IU/mL
Insulin autoantibodies	<0.4	<0.4 U/mL

TABLE 1.4　Comparing MODY to Type 1 and Type 2 Diabetes

Characteristics	MODY	T1DM	T2DM
Age at diagnosis	<25	5-25	12 – adulthood
Parental history	60%-90%	<10%	10%-14%
Inheritance	Autosomal dominant	Autoimmune	Polygenic
Obesity Insulin resistance Metabolic syndrome	Uncommon	Uncommon	Common
Beta cell Abs	Absent	Present	Absent
C-peptide	Normal	Undetectable	High to low
Optimal Tx	SU MODY[1,3,4]	Insulin	Metformin

patient would be well served to get genetic testing done to determine which type of monogenic diabetes she has, so the treatment can be as specific as possible. Maturity-onset diabetes of the young (MODY) 2 (glucokinase gene mutation) and MODY 3 (HNF-alpha mutation) are the most common forms of this condition. MODY 3 makes up about 58% of all MODY cases and MODY 2 contributes another 22%.[3] MODY 2 can be treated with a change in dietary intake with a relatively low-carbohydrate diet. MODY 3 typically is treated with a low-dose sulfonylurea.[3] The thing to know about these common types of diabetes is that there is a problem with the timing of insulin secretion, not insulin resistance or insulin deficiency.

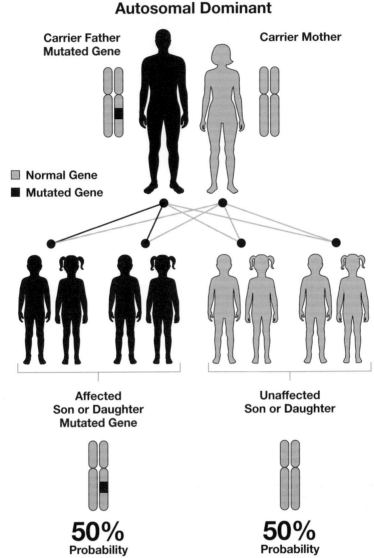

FIGURE 1.4. Autosomal dominant transmission in monogenic diabetes. *(Monogenic Diabetes (Neonatal Diabetes Mellitus & MODY).* The National Institute of Diabetes and Digestive and Kidney Diseases (NIDDK): Monogenic Diabetes. 2017. https://www.niddk. nih.gov/health-information/diabetes/overview/what-is-diabetes/monogenic-neonatal-mellitus-mody#:~:text=Neonatal%20diabetes%20mellitus%20(NDM)%20and,main%20 forms%20of%20monogenic%20diabetes)

There is an online MODY calculator to help determine if a person has MODY.[4] It is available at https://www.diabetesgenes.org/mody-probability-calculator/. To find a lab that can test for MODY, please go to: https://www.ncbi.nlm.nih.gov/gtr.[5]

Case Summary and Closing Points

MODY represents 1% of all cases of diabetes. It is a type of diabetes that is often misdiagnosed. The key to MODY is that it is an autosomal dominant condition affecting insulin production and release. People with MODY are not insulin resistant nor do they have absolute insulin deficiency. The absence of these features and the presence of a "mild" diabetes in three successive generations (diagnosed at a young age) should prompt an evaluation for MODY.

References

1. Shields BM, Hicks S, Shepherd MH, Colclough K, Hattersley AT, Ellard S. Maturity onset diabetes of the young (MODY): how many cases are we missing? *Diabetologia*. 2010;53(12):2504-2508.
2. *Monogenic Diabetes (Neonatal Diabetes Mellitus & MODY)*. The National Institute of Diabetes and Digestive and Kidney Diseases (NIDDK). 2017. https://www.niddk.nih.gov/health-information/diabetes/overview/what-is-diabetes/monogenic-neonatal-mellitus-mody#:~:text=Neonatal%20diabetes%20mellitus%20(NDM)%20and,main%20forms%20of%20monogenic%20diabetes
3. Fajans SS, Bell GI. MODY: history, genetics, pathophysiology and clinical decision making. *Diabetes Care*. 2011;34(8):1878-1884.
4. Exeter Diabetes. MODY calculator. 2022 .https://www.diabetesgenes.org/mody-probability-calculator/
5. NIH National Library of Medicine. List of MODY testing sites. 2022. https://www.ncbi.nlm.nih.gov/gtr

Case 6.   Ketosis-Prone Type 2 Diabetes

"What kind of diabetes do I have?"

A 19-year-old African American man presents to the emergency room with complaints of excessive thirst, excessive urination, and a 20-lb weight loss in the past month. He has no significant past medical history, but he does have a family history of type 2 diabetes. He does not follow any dietary plan. He gets regular exercise with an hour of basketball at least 5 d/wk.

He remembers that about 3 weeks ago he started to have excessive thirst and cravings for juices and soda but was unable to satisfy the craving. He was drinking all the time and urinating frequently day and night. His family noticed that he was losing weight and recommended that he seek medical care. Earlier, on the day of presentation, he experienced nausea and vomiting then abdominal pain, so he came to the emergency room.

He was found to be in DKA and was treated according to the hospital's DKA protocol. He required a lot of insulin over the first 48 hours and was sent home with a daily regimen of 45 units of basal insulin and 15 units per meal of mealtime (prandial) insulin. During the hospitalization, the patient's family had questions about the type of diabetes he had and how it should best be treated.

Medications: no medications, vitamins, or supplements

Allergies: no known allergies

Family Medical History: mom and dad have type 2 diabetes, hypertension, and dyslipidemia; dad has chronic kidney disease from diabetes; family history is otherwise unknown

Social History: lives at home with mom, works part time, no specific diet, get regular aerobic exercise, no tobacco, alcohol, or recreational drugs

Physical Exam: Ht. 6′1″, Wt. 229 lb, BMI 30.2, T 98.6, P 110, R 24

CV: tachycardic but no other abnormalities

RESP: tachypneic but lungs clear to auscultation

Skin: acanthosis noted on his neck and axilla

Abdomen: BS active but he has diffuse tenderness

Obese patient, currently dehydrated

 CASE QUESTIONS

1. What type of diabetes does he have? What in the case presentation confirms the diagnosis?
2. What are the initial next steps?
3. What are the long-term next steps?

ANSWERS AND EXPLANATIONS

1. Initially it is difficult to determine what type of diabetes he has.

   He is a young adult presenting in DKA, which is really the classic presentation of type 1 diabetes. However, he is obese, and he has a family history of type 2 diabetes, which significantly increases the likelihood that he actually has a form of type 2 diabetes.

2. When a patient presents in DKA, the initial treatment should be determined with the assumption that the patient has type 1 diabetes. Complete insulin replacement therapy is recommended including basal insulin and mealtime (prandial) insulin. It is also advisable to order tests to confirm the diagnosis of type 1 diabetes including measures of insulin secretion (C-peptide) and measures of autoimmunity as mentioned in Chapter 3. However, these tests are best ordered when the patient is no longer in a hyperglycemic crisis and has been stabilized with therapy. This is because anyone with severe hyperglycemia will suppress physiologic insulin secretion resulting in a low C-peptide level even though they may have preserved beta cell function under more normal glycemic status.

   This patient was treated with basal and bolus insulin therapy for 2 weeks and then asked to come back to the office. His glucose was largely within the normal range during the entire 2-week period except for two hypoglycemic episodes in the last 48 hours before his visit. He also had labs drawn prior to his outpatient visit. The results are in Table 1.5.

TABLE 1.5 Additional Labs		
Labs	**Value**	**Reference Range**
C-peptide	3.5	0.78-1.89 ng/mL (fasting)
Islet cell antibody screen	Negative	Negative
GAD antibodies	<5	<5 IU/mL
Insulin autoantibodies	<0.4	<0.4 U/mL
Lipid Panel	**Value**	**Reference Range**
Cholesterol, total	238	125-200 mg/dL
Triglycerides	180	<150 mg/dL
LDL (calculated)	164	<130 mg/dL
HDL cholesterol	38	>40 mg/dL men; >50 women
Non-HDL cholesterol	192	<130

The labs indicate that he does not have deficient insulin secretion, and he has no measures of autoimmunity. He also has traditional diabetic dyslipidemia with a low HDL and high triglycerides despite stabilization of his glucose. These findings substantially increase the likelihood that he has type 2 diabetes. If he has type 1 diabetes, it is less likely that he would have diabetic dyslipidemia or a family history of diabetes. If a definitive diagnosis cannot be ascertained, it is best to continue insulin until a final determination can be made.

There is a form of type 2 diabetes called ketosis-prone type 2 diabetes. This form of diabetes is documented more commonly in people of African descent and typically presents with DKA. This patient has a body habitus consistent with type 2 diabetes and a family history of type 2 diabetes.

Because there are more and more adults with insulin resistance who are developing type 1 diabetes, it is still important to order labs measuring insulin secretion and autoimmunity. Once the diagnosis of ketosis-prone diabetes is confirmed, patients often will be able to stop insulin once their glucose has been stabilized. It can take anywhere from 4 to 12 weeks to reach this point. It is best not to reduce insulin doses until the patient has had at least 4 weeks of stable glucose levels within the target range. Stopping insulin too soon or failing to confirm that a patient does not have markers of type 1 diabetes can result in recurrence of DKA. Late recurrence of DKA months to years later is also possible, so it is important to make sure that these patients are treated and monitored for stability.

3. Patients with ketosis-prone type 2 diabetes often can be treated with oral therapy and sometimes solely with lifestyle modification. Still, we must be vigilant in monitoring these patients knowing that if they destabilize during illnesses or experience destabilization of their lipid profiles and develop lipotoxicity, they could go back into DKA.

This patient was prescribed basal and bolus insulin for 2 weeks, reducing mealtime insulin from 15 to 8 units for 2 weeks. His glucose continued to be stable, so mealtime insulin was stopped entirely. He continued to eat a well-balanced diet and tried to limit carbohydrates to no more than 45 g/meal. His glucose continued to be near normal. He was advised to take 10 units of basal insulin off each week so that at the end of four more weeks he was no longer taking insulin. At this point, he noticed that it was harder to maintain his fasting glucose, so he was started on metformin with a titrated dose reaching 1000 mg twice a day, which he tolerated and continued to do well with.

Case Summary and Closing Points

Ketosis-prone type 2 diabetes is a form of type 2 diabetes mellitus but it often presents like type 1 diabetes. When a clinician is unsure, it is best to treat the patient as though they have type 1 until the diagnosis is clear. When a person presents with DKA but has a family history of type 2 diabetes or has phenotypical features of type 2, it is worth looking for ketosis-prone diabetes. If present, the person will not need to be on insulin for life and often can be managed with lifestyle change alone.

References

1. Umpierrez GE, Smiley D, Kitabchi AE. Narrative review: ketosis prone type 2 diabetes mellitus. *Ann Intern Med.* 2006;144(5):350-357. doi:10.7326/0003-4819-144-5-200603070-00011
2. Gaba R, Mehta P, Balasubramanyam A. Evaluation and management of ketosis-prone diabetes. *Expert Rev Endocrinol Metab.* 2019;14(1):43-48. doi:10.1080/17446651.2019.1561270

Case 7.　Pregestational Diabetes

"What do you mean I have diabetes already?"

A 29-year-old woman G3P2 at 14 weeks gestation reported to discuss her A1c. Her intake labs indicated a fasting glucose of 132 mg/dL and HbA1c at 6.9%. She reported that she did not have any history of diabetes, but that it did run in her family. She gained 10 and 15 lbs respectively with her two previous pregnancies. Both babies were delivered healthy at term (birthweights of 7 and 7 lb 6 oz).

Past Medical History: no chronic illnesses

Medications: prenatal vitamins

Allergies: none

Family Medical History: mom and dad have type 2 diabetes, hypertension, and dyslipidemia

Social History: Married in a supportive household with spouse and two children (ages 6 and 3 years). No tobacco, no alcohol, no recreational drugs. She is eating out more while trying to juggle everyone's schedules. No problem areas apparent in social determinants of health.

Physical Exam: Ht. 5'8", Wt. 199 lb, BMI 30.3, T 98.6, P 90, R 16, BP 128/76

CV: exam normal

RESP: exam normal

She is obese but in no acute distress.

Abdomen benign, gravid—appropriate for gestational age.

No other relevant abnormalities seen on testing.

 CASE QUESTIONS

1. What kind of diabetes does she have?
2. What separates pregestational diabetes from gestational diabetes?
3. What are the next steps?

 ANSWERS AND EXPLANATIONS

1. She has developed diabetes range glucose readings (both elevated fasting glucose at 132 mg/dL and HbA1c of 6.9%) at 12 weeks' gestation. Any glucose abnormality that is present prior to mid second trimester (24-28 weeks) is considered preexisting diabetes. In this case, she most likely has type 2 diabetes. Her A1c was 6.9%, which is equivalent to a mean glucose of close to 150 mg/dL over the previous 3 months.

   While she was unaware of her diabetes, she does indeed meet the diagnostic criteria. Diabetes present before the second trimester is considered a high-risk pregnancy.[1]

   It is important to note that pregestational diabetes rates have doubled since 1996 with more than 75% of those cases being preexisting type 2.[2] Further, women aged 30 or older and of African American, Hispanic, or Asian ethnicity have higher rates of preexisting type 2 diabetes.[2]

   Given her current history, it is most likely that she has preexisting type 2 pregestational diabetes.

2. The timing of identification of an abnormality in glucose metabolism separates pre-gestational diabetes (PGDM) from gestational diabetes (GDM). As discussed in the next case, GDM does not become a possibility until the middle of the second trimester when placental hormones impact insulin sensitivity enough to affect glucose metabolism. Therefore, it is recommended to test for GDM between 24 and 28 weeks' gestation.

   PGDM can be any type of preexisting diabetes present before conception up to 24 weeks' gestation. If PGDM is found before conception, patients should be encouraged to create a plan to get control of their diabetes and modify medications accordingly before conception. If the glucose abnormality is first identified during prenatal care or prior to 24 weeks during gestation, the placental hormones are not the likely cause and treatment for diabetes should start immediately.[3]

3. The HbA1c treatment goal for conception (if a woman knows she has diabetes) is 6.5%. During pregnancy, the target HbA1c is 6.0% if it can be achieved without excessive hypoglycemia.[4] All women who have diabetes (type 1, type 2, GDM)

should receive diabetes education and implement appropriate lifestyle modifications. If pharmacologic therapy is needed, it is now recommended that all women use insulin as it has the best record of efficacy and safety for both mother and fetus.[2,4]

Treatment goals during pregnancy are as follows: fasting glucose <95 mg/dL (5.3 mmol/L) and either one-hour postprandial glucose <140 mg/dL (7.8 mmol/L) or 2-hour postprandial glucose <120 mg/dL (6.7 mmol/L) with an A1c of 6.0%.[4] The insulin regimen used depends on the type of diabetes. The patient had fasting hyperglycemia and will therefore require insulin overnight. She can be treated with NPH (neutral protamine Hagedorn) at bedtime (0.1 U/kg/dose) or a long-acting basal analog insulin. Typically, insulin doses are adjusted at least weekly to help achieve target fasting glucose levels.[3]

Case Summary and Closing Points

Safety data are limited for therapeutic agents for pregnancy and planning, so it is important to rely heavily on lifestyle change and insulin (if needed) as the safety agent of choice.

Recent reports show that most US women are in poor cardiometabolic health when they get pregnant. Further, cardiometabolic complications in pregnancy predict future outcomes for both mother and baby. Therefore, it is important to distinguish PGDM from GDM. Those with PGDM will need ongoing treatment after delivery, which is not always the case with GDM.

References

1. American College of Obstetricians and Gynecologists' Committee on Practice Bulletins—Obstetrics. ACOG practice bulletin No. 201: pregestational diabetes mellitus. *Obstet Gynecol.* 2018;132(6):e228 -e248.
2. Peng TY, Ehrlich SF, Crites Y, et al. Trends and racial andethnic disparities in the prevalence of pregestational type 1and type 2 diabetes in Northern California: 1996-2014. *Am J Obstet Gynecol.* 2017;216:177. e1-177.e8.
3. Hart BN, Shubrook JH, Mason T. Pregestational diabetes and family planning. *Clin Diabetes.* 2021;39(3):323-328. doi:10.2337/cd20-0062
4. American Diabetes Association. Standards of Care for the Person with Diabetes 2022. Chapter 15: Management of Diabetes in Pregnancy. *Diabetes Care.* 2022;45(suppl 1):S232-S243. https://diabetes-journals.org/care/article/45/Supplement_1/S232/138916/15-Management-of-Diabetes-in-Pregnancy-Standards

Case 8. Gestational Diabetes

"Does this mean I need insulin?"

A 27-year-old woman who is G1P0 in her 26th week of pregnancy presented to the office to discuss her abnormal GTT. She reported that, so far, her pregnancy had been going well. It was a planned pregnancy, and she felt "pretty good." She experienced minimal nausea in her first trimester and for the last 12 weeks she has felt "pretty energetic." Her sister had diabetes during her pregnancy, so she knew she had to stay active through her pregnancy and be more careful about what she ate.

She was surprised when her GTT came back abnormal. She wants to know what she has to do now and does she really have to take insulin. She has never taken medications on a regular basis, and the prospect of doing so now is scary to her.

Past Medical History: no chronic illnesses

Medications: prenatal vitamins

Family Medical History: dad has hypertension and dyslipidemia; she had a sister who had diabetes during pregnancy, but it went away

Allergies: none

Social History: Married in a supportive household with spouse. Planned pregnancy. No tobacco, no alcohol, no recreational drugs. No problem areas apparent in social determinants of health.

Physical Exam Prepregnancy: Ht. 5′8″, Wt. 179 lb, BMI 27.2

Physical Exam Upon Presentation: Wt. 199 lb, T 98.6, P 90, R 16, BP 118/78

CV: exam normal

RESP: exam normal

She is overweight and gravid but in no acute distress.

Abdomen gravid

Extremities: trace edema lower extremities

Glucose tolerance test results: 75-g 2-hour OGTT

Fasting glucose: 90 mg/dL

1 hour: 219 mg/dL (upper limit 180 mg/dL)

2 hour: 160 mg/dL (upper limit 153 mg/dL)

 CASE QUESTIONS

1. How is gestational diabetes diagnosed?
2. What are the risk factors for gestational diabetes and its complications?
3. How is gestational diabetes managed?
4. What is recommended for screening and follow-up after delivery?
5. What is the future risk of developing type 2 diabetes in women who have had gestational diabetes?

 ANSWERS AND EXPLANATIONS

1. Gestational diabetes mellitus (GDM) is defined as new-onset hyperglycemia detected after 24 weeks' gestation. The prevalence of GDM affects 2% to 10% of pregnancies in the United States annually.[1] It is important to utilize evidence-based screening methods to allow for an early diagnosis. Diagnosing GDM is

not the same as diagnosing diabetes mellitus. GDM is diagnosed using an OGTT completed between 24 and 28 weeks' gestation. The timing of the OGTT is based upon when the placental hormonal effects are most likely to impact insulin resistance and put women at risk for GDM. Pregnancy has been coined a "diabetogenic state." This is due to the increased insulin resistance seen even in normal pregnancies secondary to the effects of human placental lactogen and progesterone.[2]

HbA1c is not used for GDM as it will not identify hyperglycemia early enough for a timely diagnosis to be made. A fasting glucose is less sensitive for diagnosis of GDM. The postprandial glucose is often the first glycemic abnormality seen in most women.[3]

There are two acceptable methods to screen for GDM,[4,5] the one-step approach and the two-step approach. A study compared the effects each on the likelihood of diagnosing GDM along with identifying pregnancy complications for mother and infant. The results showed that while the one-step approach resulted in a twofold increase in the diagnosis of GDM, it did not result in better outcomes for mothers and infants compared to the two-step approach.[6] A description of the two methods is seen in Table 1.6.[4]

TABLE 1.6 Screening Methods for Gestational Diabetes

One-step strategy

Perform a 75-g OGTT, with plasma glucose measurement when patient is fasting and at 1 and 2 h, at 24-28 wk of gestation in women not previously diagnosed with diabetes.

The OGTT should be performed in the morning after an overnight fast of at least 8 h.

The diagnosis of GDM is made when any of the following plasma glucose values are met or exceeded:

- Fasting: 92 mg/dL (5.1 mmol/L)
- 1 h: 180 mg/dL (10.0 mmol/L)
- 2 h: 153 mg/dL (8.5 mmol/L)

Two-step strategy

Step 1: Perform a 50-g GLT (nonfasting), with plasma glucose measurement at 1 h, at 24-28 wk of gestation in women not previously diagnosed with diabetes.

If the plasma glucose level measured 1 h after the load is ≥130, 135, or 140 mg/dL (7.2, 7.5, or 7.8 mmol/L, respectively), proceed to a 100-g OGTT.

Step 2: The 100-g OGTT should be performed with the patient in fasting.

The diagnosis of GDM is made when at least two[a] of the following four plasma glucose levels (measured at fasting and at 1, 2, and 3 h during OGTT) are met or exceeded (Carpenter-Coustan criteria):

- Fasting: 95 mg/dL (5.3 mmol/L)
- 1 h: 180 mg/dL (10.0 mmol/L)
- 2 h: 155 mg/dL (8.6 mmol/L)
- 3 h: 140 mg/dL (7.8 mmol/L)

GDM, gestational diabetes mellitus; GLT, glucose load test; OGTT, oral glucose tolerance test.

American Diabetes Association Professional Practice Committee. 2. Classification and Diagnosis of Diabetes: Standards of Medical Care in Diabetes—2022. *Diabetes Care.* 2022;45(suppl 1):S17-S38. https://doi.org/10.2337/dc22-S002

[a]The American College of Obstetricians and Gynecologists notes that one elevated value can be used for diagnosis.

2. As previously mentioned, circulating placental hormones are responsible for creating a diabetogenic state.[2,7] GDM is high risk when the following risk factors are
present: increasing maternal age, family history of diabetes/prediabetes, preconception obesity, excessive weight gain prior to and throughout pregnancy, and
long-term barriers to health care (aka socioeconomic disparities).[8]

   Unmanaged GDM leads to poor health outcomes in both mother and
infant.[9,10] Maternal risks include preeclampsia, preterm labor, and a sevenfold
increased risk of developing maternal type 2 diabetes mellitus.[10] Fetal health
is compromised by intrauterine exposure to persistent hyperglycemia and can
result in macrosomia, hypoglycemia, and perinatal complications including
preterm delivery and fetal demise, as well as future obesity and insulin resistance
in the fetus.[10]

3. The management of GDM starts with a timely diagnosis. Once GDM is confirmed,
referral to a dietitian and the introduction of diabetes education are essential. Note
that many women are able to normalize glucose readings with lifestyle changes
alone[11] (Table 1.7).[11,12]

   If the patient is not able to achieve the above glucose goals with lifestyle changes,
pharmacotherapy is recommended. The American Diabetes Association currently
recommends that all women who require treatment for GDM or pregnancy complicated by diabetes should manage glucose with insulin-based therapeutic regimens.[11] This is because other medications such as sulfonylureas and metformin
have been shown to cross the placenta and may have adverse outcomes for the
fetus.[11]

   For many women, achieving normal fasting glucose is the biggest challenge.
For this reason, a long-acting basal insulin analog or insulin NPH given at bedtime is usually the first step to treatment. If postprandial hyperglycemia occurs,
then a mealtime insulin regimen is also suggested.

Case Summary and Closing Points

Gestational diabetes (GDM) is increasing in frequency and severity. It is important for
clinicians to recognize that GDM increases a women's future risk of type 2 diabetes by
as much as 58% and can increase a baby's risk for type 2 diabetes. The role of the primary care provider is to encourage postpartum diabetes screening, breast feeding, and
a healthy postpregnancy weight.

TABLE 1.7	Glucose Targets in Women With Gestational Diabetes		
Fasting	**1-h Postprandial**	**2-h Postprandial**	**HbA1c**
<95 mg/dL (5.3 mmol/L)	<140 mg/dL (7.8 mmol/L)	<120 mg/dL (6.7 mmol/L)	<6.0%

American Diabetes Association. Standards of Care for the Person with Diabetes 2022. Chapter15: Management of Diabetes
in Pregnancy. *Diabetes Care*. 2022;45(suppl 1):S232-S243. https://diabetesjournals.org/care/article/45/Supplement_1/
S232/138916/15-Management-of-Diabetes-in-Pregnancy-Standards. Metzger BE, Buchanan TA, Coustan DR, et al. Summary and
recommendations of the Fifth International Workshop-Conference on Gestational Diabetes Mellitus. *Diabetes Care*. 2007;30(suppl
2):S251-S260. doi:10.2337/dc07-s225.

References

1. Sheiner E. Gestational diabetes mellitus: long-term consequences for the mother and child grand challenge—how to move on towards secondary prevention? *Front Clin Diabet Health.* 2020;1:543256. doi:10.3389/fcdhc.2020.546256

2. Gabbe SG, Graves CR. Management of diabetes mellitus complicating pregnancy. *Obstet Gynecol.* 2003;102(4):857-868.

3. McIntyre HD, Sacks DA, Barbour LA, et al. Issues with the diagnosis and classification of hyperglycemia in early pregnancy. *Diabetes Care.* 2016;39(1):53-54. doi:10.2337/dc15-1887

4. American Diabetes Association Professional Practice Committee; 2. Classification and diagnosis of diabetes: Standards of medical care in diabetes—2022. *Diabetes Care* 2022; 45(suppl 1):S17-S38. doi:10.2337/dc22-S002

5. Mack LR, Tomich PG. Gestational diabetes: diagnosis, classification, and clinical care. *Obstet Gynecol Clin North Am.* 2017;44(2):207-217. doi:10.1016/j.ogc.2017.02.002

6. Hillier TA, Pedula KL, Ogasawara KK, et al. A pragmatic, randomized clinical trial of gestational diabetes screening. *N Engl J Med.* 2021;384(10):895-904. doi:10.1056/NEJMoa2026028

7. Plows JF, Stanley JL, Baker PN, Reynolds CM, Vickers MH. The pathophysiology of gestational diabetes mellitus. *Int J Mol Sci.* 2018;19(11):3342. doi:10.3390/ijms19113342

8. Ha C, Shubrook JH, Mason T. Gestational diabetes: optimizing diagnosis and management in primary care. *J Fam Pract.* 2022;71(2):2-9.

9. Angueira AR, Ludvik AE, Reddy TE, Wicksteed B, Lowe WL, Jr., Layden BT. New insights into gestational glucose metabolism: lessons learned from 21st century approaches. *Diabetes.* 2015;64(2):327-334. doi:10.2337/db14-0877

10. Shou C, Wei YM, Wang C, et al. Updates in long-term maternal and fetal adverse effects of gestational diabetes mellitus. *Maternal-Fetal.* 2019;1:91-94. doi:10.1097/FM9.0000000000000019

11. American Diabetes Association. Standards of Care for the Person with Diabetes 2022. Chapter15: Management of Diabetes in Pregnancy. *Diabetes Care.* 2022;45(suppl 1):S232-S243. https://diabetesjournals.org/care/article/45/Supplement_1/S232/138916/15-Management-of-Diabetes-in-Pregnancy-Standards

12. Metzger BE, Buchanan TA, Coustan DR, et al. Summary and recommendations of the Fifth International Workshop-conference on gestational diabetes mellitus. *Diabetes Care.* 2007;30(suppl 2):S251-S260. doi:10.2337/dc07-s225

Case 9. Secondary Diabetes

"Why did I get diabetes?"

A 54-year-old woman presented for follow-up after a hospital visit. Her initial complaint was 2 weeks of abdominal pain, nausea, vomiting, and smelly and greasy bowel movements. She was diagnosed with acute pancreatitis but was also found to have hyperglycemia. She had no personal or family history of diabetes. She was in the hospital for 4 days.

She reported no known medical issues. The only medications she reported taking were antacids and OTC proton pump inhibitors for an upset stomach. Her chart revealed she had had at least 2 previous episodes of pancreatitis in the past 5 years that required hospitalization.

Past Medical History: no chronic illnesses

Medications: Tums, OTC omeprazole prn

Family Medical History: Significant for chronic alcohol use in her father. Mother had colon cancer. Both are deceased. She has a sister, but she is not aware of her medical history.

Allergies: none

Social History: She is currently employed at a convenience store. She does not smoke but does binge drink periodically—usually with vodka and 12 pack of beer. However, she has not had a drink since she left the hospital. She lives alone and has a pet cat. Diet is largely snack foods. She does not get any regular exercise outside of work.

Physical Exam: Ht. 5'6", Wt. 130 lb, BMI 21, T 98.6, P 102, R 16

She appears nervous but in no acute distress.

CV: exam normal

RESP: exam normal

Abdomen: not currently tender, but hepatomegaly is noted

Extremities: normal

A1c at hospital 8 weeks ago: 8.6%

A1c at today's visit: 9.8%

Lab Values:

Lipid Panel	Value	Reference Range
Cholesterol, total	188	125-200 mg/dL
Triglycerides	60	<150 mg/dL
LDL (calculated)	92	<130 mg/dL
HDL cholesterol	74	>40 mg/dL men; >50 women
Non-HDL cholesterol	108	<130

Additional Labs	Value	Reference Range
C-peptide	0.6	0.78-1.89 ng/mL (fasting)
Islet cell antibody screen	Negative	Negative
GAD antibodies	<5	<5 IU/mL
Insulin autoantibodies	<0.4	<0.4 U/mL

Comprehensive Metabolic Panel	Value	Reference Range
Sodium	141	136-145 mmol/L
Potassium, serum	4.2	3.5-5.3 mmol/L
Chloride, serum	99	98-110 mmol/L
Carbon dioxide (CO_2)	26	19-30 mmol/L
Urea nitrogen, blood (BUN)	15	7-25 mg/dL
Creatinine, serum	0.64	0.5-1.10 mg/dL
eGFR	104	>60 mL/min/1.73 m^2
Glucose, serum	225	65-99 mg/dL
Calcium, serum	9.9	8.6-10.2 mg/dL

Comprehensive Metabolic Panel	Value	Reference Range
Protein, total	6.0.3	6.1-8.1 g/dL
Albumin	3.6	3.6-4.1 g/dL
Globulin	2.8	1.9-3.7 g/dL
AST (SGOT)	164	10-35 U/L
ALT (SGPT)	138	6-29 U/L
Bilirubin, total	1.4	0.2-1.2 mg/dL
Alkaline phosphatase	100	33-115 U/L

Pancreatic Tests	Result	Normal Range
Amylase	68	40-140 U/L
Lipase	160	10-140 U/L

CBC:

CBC	Value	Reference Range
White blood cell count	8.8	3.8-10.8 thousand/µL
Red blood cell count	3.8	3.8-5.10 million/µL
Hemoglobin	12.9	12.6-17 g/dL
Hematocrit	40	37%-51%
MCV	91	80-100 fL
MCH	29.9	27-33 pg
MCHC	32.9	32-36 g/dL
RDW	12.7	1%-15%
Platelet count	138	140-400 thousand/µL
Basophils	1	%
Bands	0	0%-10%

 CASE QUESTIONS

1. Does she have diabetes? If so, what type?
2. How is this type of diabetes different from type 1 and type 2?
3. What are the next steps?

 ANSWERS AND EXPLANATIONS

1. The patient had abdominal pain but no "poly" symptoms when she presented with pancreatitis. While pancreatitis can cause hyperglycemia during an acute episode, this patient is feeling better but still has hyperglycemia and a low C-peptide. Therefore, she meets the diagnostic criteria for diabetes mellitus and likely has secondary diabetes.[1]

Secondary diabetes makes up a small percentage of total diabetes cases. It is important to find the cause and make an accurate diagnosis to address the underlying pathophysiology. The most common etiologies of secondary diabetes include chronic pancreatitis (79%), pancreatic ductal carcinoma (8%), hemochromatosis (7%), cystic fibrosis (4%), and previous pancreatic surgery (2%).[2]

2. Remember from previous cases that type 1 diabetes typically presents with the "polys" and weight loss. Many patients will present in DKA. People with type 1 typically have no family history of diabetes but will often have a personal or family history of autoimmune disease. The most common lab findings are a low C-peptide (with glucose >144 mg/dL—must be ordered together) and often markers of autoimmunity.

Type 2 diabetes most often is "discovered" from laboratory screening. While patients may not have any symptoms, they usually have a family history of diabetes/prediabetes and will often have an elevated BMI indicative of increased body weight. The most common indicative lab finding is diabetic dyslipidemia represented by high triglycerides and low HDL. It is usually unnecessary to obtain a C-peptide in patients newly diagnosed with type 2 diabetes. However, if ordered, most asymptomatic patients with type 2 diabetes will have a normal to high C-peptide with a normal to high glucose. These tests should not be ordered during a hyperglycemic crisis in which glucose toxicity will alter the results.

This patient was found to have hyperglycemia upon admission to the hospital. Even after the acute illness resolved, her hyperglycemia continued. Once this acute illness resolved, her hyperglycemic persisted and her HbA1c indicated that she had chronic hyperglycemia and established a diagnosis of diabetes. She did not have obesity (BMI > 30) or diabetes-related dyslipidemia (making type 2 less likely). She also had a slightly depressed C-peptide and no measures of autoimmunity.

Given these factors, a provisional diagnosis of secondary diabetes makes sense based upon her presentation.

3. Secondary diabetes is a form of diabetes that occurs when the patient is insulinopenic, but the etiology is not as a result of autoimmunity. Rather, something else is causing beta cell failure. In this patient's case, alcohol-induced pancreatitis is the likely etiology.

Since the patient is insulinopenic, insulin must be part of the treatment plan. Most patients with secondary diabetes will end up with treatments similar to patients with type 1 diabetes. However, since this particular patient does not have an autoimmune condition, special attention should be paid to the etiology and management of the underlying condition. This patient does not have type 1 diabetes, and therefore, no other routine autoimmune screenings are needed.

Case Summary and Closing Points

As outlined above, there are many different types and causes of diabetes. Secondary diabetes is unique in that it is not autoimmune, not from insulin resistance, and not an inherited condition but rather the result of some other process that is harming the pancreas' ability to secret insulin. This can often come from anatomic or biochemical destruction of the pancreas. In this case, the damage from alcohol-induced pancreatitis caused insulin deficiency. Secondary diabetes is treated with insulin.

References

1. American Diabetes Association Professional Practice Committee. 2. Classification and diagnosis of diabetes: Standards of medical care in diabetes—2022. *Diabetes Care.* 2022;45(suppl 1):S17-S38. doi:10.2337/dc22-S002

2. Hart PA, Bellin MD, Andersen DK, et al; Consortium for the Study of Chronic Pancreatitis, Diabetes, and Pancreatic Cancer (CPDPC). Type 3c (pancreatogenic) diabetes mellitus secondary to chronic pancreatitis and pancreatic cancer. *Lancet Gastroenterol Hepatol.* 2016;1(3):226-237. ISSN 2468-1253. doi:10.1016/S2468-1253(16)30106-6

Initial Approach to the Patient

Introduction

Receiving a diagnosis of diabetes is life changing and usually overwhelming. Helping patients get off to a strong start and establishing a treatment plan for success can make all the difference for both the patient and the clinician. This chapter explores how to initiate treatment plans for adults and children diagnosed with diabetes, with special attention to key aspects of education, early intensive treatments, and the benefits of a team-based approach.

Case 1. Type 2 Adult

"Step-down therapy is better than step-up therapy."

A 62-year-old man presents for a diabetes follow-up. He has type 2 diabetes (10 years), hypertension (12 years), and dyslipidemia (10 years). Unfortunately, he missed his last two scheduled appointments. You recall he was previously actively involved in managing his diabetes, and it had been well-controlled. He tells you today that his diabetes medications are no longer working. His blood sugars are always above 200 mg/dL and at times, after meals his meter just reads "high." He stopped doing fingerstick glucose readings because he got frustrated by how high his readings were.

He has been using the same diabetes medications for the past 2 years. He acknowledges feeling more depressed and anxious because his readings are so high. He does not understand why diabetes is different from hypertension. He has been on the same blood pressure medications for a long time, and his blood pressure has always been controlled.

Past Medical History: hypertension, type 2 diabetes, dyslipidemia, knee osteoarthritis (OA)

Medications: metformin 1000 mg bid, glipizide 10 mg bid, sitagliptin 100 mg daily, atorvastatin 40 mg daily, lisinopril HCTZ 20/25 mg daily, amlodipine 5 mg daily, meloxicam 15 mg daily

Allergies: none

Family Medical History: parents deceased: mom—old age, dad—myocardial infarction (MI); two older brothers with similar health problems

Social History: lives alone (divorced 6 months ago); two adult children; breakfast is often coffee and a pastry; lunch is fast food 50% of time; dinner is preprepared meals; prior to his divorce, his wife cooked meals at home. He works for the public utilities service and is active on his job; no other regular physical activity. No tobacco, rarely alcohol.

Physical Exam

Vitals: HR 72, R 14, BP 136/82, Ht. 66 inches, Wt. 204 lb, BMI 32.9

General: truncal obesity

CV: normal

Resp: normal

EXT: pulses intact, monofilament, and vibration sensation intact. Skin and nails
    normal

Exam otherwise normal

Lab Values:

Lipid Panel	Value	Reference Range
Cholesterol, total	208	125-200 mg/dL
Triglycerides	256	<150 mg/dL
LDL (calculated)	108	<130 mg/dL
HDL, cholesterol	32	>40 mg/dL men; >50 women
Non-HDL cholesterol	178	<130

Other Labs	Value	Reference Range
HbA1c	9.2%	<5.7% (normal)
Urine albumin/creatinine ratio (UACr)	20 mg/g	<30 mg/g
Estimated glomerular filtration rate (eGFR)	88 mL/min	>60 mL/min/1.73 m²

 CASE QUESTIONS

1. How to approach this patient?
2. What to suggest in terms of glycemic management?
3. How to prevent this scenario in the first place?
4. What are the options for early intensive therapy?

ANSWERS AND EXPLANATIONS

1. What this patient is describing is a very common scenario. Type 2 diabetes is a
   chronic, progressive condition. The medications we use are intended to improve
   glycemia and reduce the risk of complications. However, current approaches to
   care do little to address the natural history and underlying pathophysiology of the
   disease state. As a result, patients often require modifications to their medication
   regimen over time (see box "Adding Diabetes Medications").

   The demands of successfully living with diabetes can be extremely challenging.
   Not uncommonly patients become frustrated and depressed when, despite their
   best efforts, their blood sugar readings are higher than desired. Often, in response
   patients will stop trying to manage their diabetes. They no longer perform

fingerstick glucose readings and may stray from their diet. Many people find that the work of taking care of their diabetes has become too overwhelming.

For this patient, the first step is to normalize his experience. We can acknowledge the patient's frustration that he continues to take his medication but does not necessarily see the benefit. Most diabetes medications (including the ones he is taking) will lose their efficacy over time. In addition, his diet has changed considerably since his divorce. Therefore, it is not surprising that his glucose levels have been climbing.

The next step is to help him gain a better understanding of what is going on with his diabetes while not overwhelming him with too much information. There is some good news that could be shared with this patient. Despite having had diabetes for more than 10 years, he does not appear to have any diabetes-related complications. This can likely be attributed to his prior excellent self-management behaviors. Bringing attention to these factors is a good way to start the visit, reminding the patient that he can still prevent complications by effectively managing his diabetes.

This might also be a good time to speak with the patient about what his goals are and what is most important to him. This allows for greater patient engagement; having him identify his treatment priorities promotes ownership over aspects directly affecting his care. Establishing a locus of control with shared decision making enhances the likelihood that the patient will adhere to his treatment plan. One approach to accomplish this is to use a patient handout with itemized goals and a checklist of "to do" items that can help him understand the overall treatment strategy. Below are examples of checklists (see boxes "How Often Should I Check My Blood Sugar?" "Blood Sugar Goals," and "Other Treatment Goals").

How Often Should I Check My Blood Sugar?_____ **times per day**
__X_ First thing in the <u>morning</u> before you eat or drink and at bedtime
_____ Before lunch or dinner
__X_ Whenever you feel that your blood sugar is low (experiencing symptoms)
__X_ Always check before you take a shot of insulin

My basal insulin is _____. My dose is _____units at _____ time.
My mealtime and correction scale insulin is _____. I take _____ units for my food 15 or 30 minutes BEFORE breakfast, lunch, dinner (circle time before and meals).

My correction scale is:	__0_ units if less than 150
	_____ units if glucose 151-200
	_____ units if glucose 201-250
	_____ units if glucose 251-300
	_____ units if glucose 301-350
	_____ units if glucose greater than 351

I also take: _____

Blood Sugar Goals	
A1C blood sugar average over 3 mo	Less than　6.5%　7%　7.5%　8%
Blood sugar <u>before</u> eating	80-130 mg/dL or _____mg/dL
Blood sugar 2 h <u>after</u> a meal	Less than 180 mg/dL or _____mg/dL

Other Treatment Goals	
Blood pressure	Less than 130/80 mm Hg or 140/90 mm Hg
Aspirin	All people at 50 years or older with cardiovascular disease (CVD) and low risk of bleeding
Statin (based on age and risk of heart attack and stroke in the next 10 years and LDL level)	High intensity Moderate intensity None

Screenings			
Annual "Comprehensive" Foot Exam	Yes	No	Date:
Foot should be assessed at each diabetes care visit			
Annual Eye Exam	Yes	No	Date:
Subsequent examinations for type 1 and type 2 patients with diabetes should be repeated annually by an ophthalmologist or optometrist			
Annual Lipid Screening	Yes	No	Date:
Annual Liver (Liver Function Test) Screening	Yes	No	Date:
Annual Test for Kidney Function	Yes	No	Date:
Urine albumin and eGFR in type 1 patients with diabetes duration of ≥5 years, in all type 2 patients with diabetes, and in all patients with comorbid hypertension starting at diagnosis			
How often should I get my A1C checked?		6 mo	3 mo
A1C well controlled, then check every 6 mo			
A1C not at goal or ≥ 7%, then check every 3 mo			
Routine Blood Pressure Readings	Yes	No	
Blood pressure should be measured at every routine diabetes visit. Patients found to have systolic blood pressure ≥140 or diastolic blood pressure ≥90 mm Hg.			

Medications		
Should I be on aspirin therapy?	Yes	No
Consider aspirin therapy (75-162 mg/d) as a primary prevention strategy in those with type 1 or type 2 diabetes • Increased cardiovascular risk (10-year risk >10%) • Men or women aged 50 years or older • At least one additional major risk factor (family history of CVD, hypertension, smoking, dyslipidemia, or albuminuria)		
Should I be on statin therapy?	Yes	No
≥ 40 years of age, CVD, or CVD risk factors include LDL cholesterol ≥100 mg/dL, high blood pressure, smoking, and overweight, and obesity; <40 years of age with additional ASCVD risk factors.		

Vaccinations			
Annual Flu Vaccine	Yes	No	Date:
≥6 months of age			
Pneumococcal Vaccine	Yes	No	Date:
Administer pneumococcal polysaccharide vaccine 23 (PPSV23) to all patients with diabetes ≥2 years of age.			
Adults ≥ 65 years of age, if not previously vaccinated, should receive pneumococcal conjugate vaccine 13 (PCV13), followed by PPSV23 6 to 12 months after initial vaccination.			
Adults ≥ 65 years of age, if previously vaccinated with PPSV23, should receive a follow-up ≥ 12 mo with PCV13.			
Hepatitis B Vaccination	Yes	No	
Administer hepatitis B vaccination to unvaccinated adults with diabetes who are aged 19 to 59 years.			

It is important to give this patient hope so that he can regain a sense of control. Type 2 diabetes is largely self-managed. One study estimated that 95% of all diabetes-related management is completed by the patient.[1] Another study surveyed certified diabetic educators to estimate the amount of time needed daily to complete diabetes self-care tasks. The results showed that comprehensive diabetes self-care can take more than 3 h/d for type 2 diabetes, and up to 5 h/d for type 1 diabetes.[2]

Because diabetes is largely self-managed, it is important that patients are well versed in the skills necessary to complete their self-care tasks. Prior to his divorce, it is possible that his spouse may have had a role in managing some of his diabetes care. Now he will need to assume responsibility for those tasks. Clearly this patient is no longer confident in his ability to effectively manage his diabetes. Because he is struggling, it may be beneficial to help him set small goals at first to help build his confidence and regain his self-efficacy. For example, by reinforcing effective self-management skills we can help him move from viewing his glucose monitoring as a threat to a tool he can use to promote positive behaviors.

The American Diabetes Association (ADA), in its Standards of Care, recommends an assessment every 3 to 6 months of the patient's achievement toward shared glucose targets and, if they are not at goal, consideration of further intensification of treatment.[3] While this may sound simple, it is anything but. Visits with a health care professional are typically rather short. Too often, providers forget to acknowledge the work of managing diabetes as opposed to focusing on just the metrics.

Diabetes self-management education and support are critical components to help our patients acquire the necessary skills to successfully manage their diabetes. This is often best accomplished via support from other members of the patient's medical team. This might include a dietician, diabetes educator, or pharmacist. The ADA currently recommends people receive diabetes education at the time of diagnosis; at the time of any major change in their health, including diabetes-related complications; anytime a change in life occurs such as divorce, death, or change in self-care responsibilities; and at any change in treatment such as the initiation of injectable therapies.

Similarly, diabetes care guidelines recommend screening for psychosocial issues (ie, diabetes distress, depression, anxiety, eating disorders) at the time of these major changes in health and/or life. For this particular patient, screening for diabetes distress and depression makes the most sense. During his diabetes recheck, he said that he thought his meds were no longer working. He stopped checking his sugars because he was upset when he saw the high numbers. He also mentioned that he did not understand the difference between managing his hypertension and his diabetes. His comments suggest frustration with self-management, which can be a major contributor to moderate to severe levels of diabetes distress. Additionally, screening for depression is recommended given that he lives alone, was divorced 2 years ago, and is 62 years old. Older adults are two to four times more likely to have depression than the general population, and they account for nearly one-fifth of suicides (18%) in the United States. The most common risk factors for suicide in older adults include loss of a loved one, social isolation and loneliness, major life changes (eg, divorce, retirement), physical illness (eg, diabetes, chronic pain), and poor perceived health. This patient shows signs that he is at risk for depression and suicide.

Importantly, screening does not need to take a lot of time. There are brief, validated measures for diabetes distress and depression (see Table 2.1).

TABLE 2.1   Brief, Validated Measures of Diabetes Distress and Depression

Measure	Items	Time to Complete	Scoring	Cost	Citation
Problem Areas in Diabetes 5 (PAID-5)	5	1-2 minutes	Scores are summed, generating a total score between 0 and 20. A score ≥8 is indicative of high distress. Individual items rated as "serious problem" are worthy of clinical attention even if score is <8.	No cost; available online	McGuire BE, Morrison TG, Hermanns N, et al. Short-form measures of diabetes-related emotional distress: the Problem Areas in Diabetes Scale (PAID)-5 and PAID-1. *Diabetologia*. 2010;53(1):66-9. doi:10.1007/s00125-009-1559-5.[4]
Problem Areas in Diabetes 1 (PAID-1)	1	1 minute	A score ≥3 is indicative of high distress.	No cost; available online	McGuire BE, Morrison TG, Hermanns N, et al. Short-form measures of diabetes-related emotional distress: the Problem Areas in Diabetes Scale (PAID)-5 and PAID-1. *Diabetologia*. 2010;53(1):66-9. doi:10.1007/s00125-009-1559-5.[4]
Diabetes Distress Scale 2 (DDS-2)	2	1 minute	Items are averaged or summed. An average ≥ 3 or sum ≥6 indicates moderate to high diabetes distress.	No cost; available online	Fisher L, Glasgow RE, Mullan JT, Skaff MM, Polonsky WH. Development of a brief diabetes distress screening instrument. *Ann Fam Med*. 2008;6(3):246-52. doi:10.1370/afm.842.[5]
Patient Health Questionnaire-2 (PHQ-2)	2	1 minute	A score ≥ 3 is the recommended cut point.	No cost; available online	

2. The current ADA treatment algorithm provides recommendations for the use of medication in the treatment of type 2 diabetes (see the table in the ADA Standards of Medical Care 2022 hyperglycemia treatment algorithm[3]). While it looks rather complicated, breaking this algorithm into small sections can make it much more straightforward.

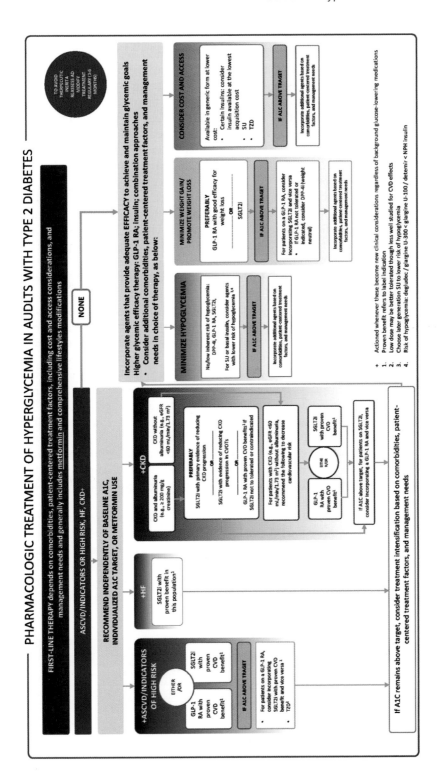

Let us start with the blue box on the very top left in the ADA Standards of Medical Care 2022 hyperglycemia treatment algorithm.[3] The most important thing to take from this is that every patient should have comprehensive diabetes self-management education and support at the time of diagnosis. Health care professionals often do not have the time or expertise to take a deep dive into therapeutic lifestyle changes for their patients. With short visits, patients often will not have the opportunity to ask all their questions of their health care providers. Dedicated time is necessary to cover the key aspects of diabetes self-care. Therefore, an early referral for diabetes education is critically important to help patients get their questions answered with meaningful information, so they can succeed in diabetes self-management.

The next step on the ADA algorithm is the red box on the left. Most patients will be initiated on metformin. It is important to determine whether a patient has a compelling indication(s), for example, atherosclerotic cardiovascular disease (ASCVD), heart failure, and kidney disease, for very specific therapies. If the patient has one or more of these conditions, treatment will coincide with the left side of the algorithm. Our patient in this case presentation does not have any of these conditions. The next step is to consult the right side of the algorithm.

Then we can ask the patient about their priorities in terms of treatment goals and concerns they may have with their current medications. Typically, issues such as undesired side effects, weight gain, hypoglycemia, and expense take precedent. This approach gives the patient the opportunity to express their priorities and enables the provider to make suggestions that will match those priorities.

The patient's A1c = 9.2%; his diabetes is no longer on target on his current regimen. He has been using metformin, a DPP4 inhibitor, and a sulfonylurea (SU).

It is important to recognize that metformin and SUs will lose efficacy over time. Metformin has a 40% failure rate at 5 years—this failure rate is higher if metformin is not started at diagnosis.[7] With SUs, about 20% of people will not respond to them due to a lack of functioning beta cells. Further, about 5% of people on SUs will stop responding to them—leaving a <u>50% nonresponder rate at 6 years</u>[8] and most will not respond to a SU at 10 years.

The options at this point include a basal insulin, a GLP-1 receptor agonist, or a SGLT-2 inhibitor. Since the patient does not have a compelling indication, each option is reasonable. Shared decision making is important at this step. The patient may have strong preferences about performing injections versus taking more oral medications. Other considerations may be side-effect profiles, whether the medication may promote weight gain or weight loss, and how quickly the treatment will work, medication expense, and insurance coverage.

Adding Diabetes Medications

Class	Agent	Instructions
GLP-1 (glucagon-like peptide 1) receptor agonists	Victoza (liraglutide)	Week 1: 0.6 mg daily Week 2: 1.2 mg daily Week 3 and thereafter: 1.8 mg daily

Class	Agent	Instructions
	Trulicity (dulaglutide)	Weeks 1 and 2: 0.75 mg weekly Week 3 and thereafter: 1.5 mg weekly *Can increase to 3.0 and 4.5 mg if needed*
	Ozempic (semaglutide)	Weeks 1-4: 0.25 mg weekly Weeks 5-8 (or longer): 0.5 mg weekly
	Rybelsus (oral semaglutide)	*Can increase to 1 or 2 mg weekly if needed* 3 mg daily on empty stomach and 4 oz of water for 30 days, then 7 mg daily *Can increase to 14 mg daily if needed (after 30 days of 7 mg)*
	Bydureon (exenatide—weekly)	2 mg once weekly at any time of day
	Byetta (exenatide—twice daily)	5 mcg twice daily before meals within 60 minutes *Can increase to 10 μg twice daily after 1 month of 5 μg*
Dual GLP/GIP (glucose-dependent insulino-tropic polypeptide) receptor agonists	Mounjaro (tirzepatide)	2.5 mg weekly *Can increase 2.5 mg/wk every 4 weeks if needed*
SGLT-2 (sodium-glucose cotransporter 2) inhibitors	Jardiance (empagliflozin)	Once daily
	Invokana (canagliflozin)	*Pay attention to urinary tract infection symptoms and keep yourself hydrated*
	Farxiga (dapagliflozin)	
	Steglatro (ertugliflozin)	
DPP-4 (dipeptidyl pepti-dase 4) inhibitors	Nesina (alogliptin)	Once daily
	Onglyza (saxagliptin)	*Not recommended to be used with GLP-1 RA*
	Tradjenta (linagliptin)	
	Januvia (sitagliptin)	
Insulin	Insulin N (NPH)	Basal/background insulin _____ units
	Toujeo (glargine)	Can be taken at bedtime <u>OR</u> in the morning
	Tresiba (degludec)	
	Basaglar (glargine)	
	Lantus (glargine)	
	Semglee (glargine-yfgn)	
	Levemir (detemir)	

Class	Agent	Instructions
	Insulin R (regular)	Bolus/mealtime insulin _____ units
	Novolog (aspart)	Inject 15 or 30 minutes before a meal (1 to 3 times daily)
	Humalog (lispro)	
	Apidra (glulisine)	
	Fiasp (aspart)	Bolus/mealtime insulin _____ units
	Lyumjev (lispro-aabc)	Inject right before OR within 20 minutes of a meal (1 to 3 times daily)
Fixed ratio injections	Soliqua (glargine + lixisenatide) Xultophy (degludec + liraglutide)	Start 16 units daily Start 15 units daily

Basal insulin is the most potent medication, but it can increase the risk of hypoglycemia and weight gain. GLP-1RAs have good fasting and postprandial coverage and will likely result in significant weight loss. They are currently formulated as once-weekly injections, once- or twice-daily injections, or a single daily oral tablet. For many patients that are reluctant to perform injections, a once-weekly administration may be an acceptable option. Our patient would need to discontinue his DPP4i if he were to start a GLP1a as they have similar mechanisms of action. The SGLT-2 inhibitors are less potent than the other agents, but are taken orally, are less expensive than the GLP-1RAs, and have the added potential to improve blood pressure levels. Even though the SU is no longer effective, it is prudent to add a treatment before reducing or stopping the SU.

When starting a new diabetes agent, it is important to share with patients what they can expect in terms of changes in blood glucose. For example, if the patient is started on basal insulin, they should know they will need to monitor their morning glucose for its effect and to help adjust their insulin dose.

At this visit, the clinician can discuss the utility of fingerstick glucose monitoring or use of a continuous glucose monitoring (CGM) system to test the efficacy of the new treatment. Some providers may have the ability to offer an office-based CGM system for short-term use. A CGM system can be a very powerful tool to help the patient see "how their life affects their diabetes."

Once a treatment plan has been agreed on and implemented, it is important to bring the patient back within 2 to 4 weeks for follow-up. He will be making major regimen changes including new medication, resumption of glucose monitoring, dietary modification, and will have received diabetes self-management education and support. Close follow-up provides an opportunity to evaluate the effectiveness of the regimen change, problem-solve if necessary, and provide encouragement. This is particularly relevant when the work of change is great.

No matter what treatment is recommended, it is key to bring the patient back at least every 3 months to reassess progress made toward reaching goals and to identify any barriers that get in the way. It has been shown that the more visits a person has specific to their diabetes the better the control they have.[9]

Another important thing to remember is to ask patients open-ended questions at these follow-up visits. This allows the patient to verbalize feelings and provide information in their own words. Next, employ active listening skills via reflection, or repeating statements back to the patient in the tone of a question, and summarizing, or recapping the patient's conversation, to show the patient that you have been listening. It also presents an opportunity to correct any misunderstandings between the two of you. Perhaps most importantly, reflecting and summarizing communicate empathy to your patient, and patients with type 2 diabetes who experience higher levels of empathy from their physician show a 40%-50% lower risk of all-cause mortality 10 years later.

3. Historically, when people were diagnosed with type 2 diabetes, they were initially advised to make lifestyle changes and then return in 3 months to see if they required medication. The great majority of these people needed to make substantial lifestyle changes and did not have the tools or guidance to understand what changes were essential. Typically, most people would be prescribed medications when they returned in 3 months. One can only imagine the frustration of those people who did make significant efforts still being told they would need to start medication, leading them to assume that lifestyle changes are not effective in the management of diabetes.

The 2022 ADA guidelines recommend starting BOTH therapeutic lifestyle changes and pharmacotherapy at diagnosis. As mentioned earlier, delaying metformin initiation even 3 months after diagnosis reduces the benefit of this medication. In fact, one study showed that starting metformin 3 months after diagnosis reduced the durability by 56%.[8]

Ralph DeFronzo, MD, labeled typical diabetes care as "treat to fail" practices.[10] Following the conventional treatment guidelines of the times, providers waited until a patient's glucose was out of control before adding medication. This approach created a situation where glucose regulation was never maintained for any length of time. Consequently, providers continually added more medication to catch up with the glucose levels without ever establishing long-term control.

Rather than following this "step-up therapy," it may be prudent to aggressively treat the condition at diagnosis, establish glycemic control with multiple modalities, and then use "step-down therapy." Despite several studies having shown this approach to be successful, it still has not become common practice. By using "step-down therapy" to achieve euglycemia, we are more likely to increase patient confidence that they can get control of their condition. This is especially true when there is a "legacy effect" of early intensive treatment with a reduction in numbers and dosages of medications used over time, versus increasing medication which is the more typical patient experience.

Research has shown that some of these early intensive initial therapies have helped put diabetes into "remission." Remission is defined as a minimum of 6 months of normal glycemic control with a HbA1c less than 6.5% with no pharmacologic therapy. One meta-analysis found that after 2 to 4 weeks of intensive therapy, 59% of people were in remission at 6 months and 46% were in remission at 1 year.[8] There is growing evidence that the timing and approach to early intensive therapy is critically important. For example, numerous studies have shown that early intensive insulin therapy can induce diabetes remission.[8-22] Another study by this team found that providing this intervention in the first 2 years of diagnosis is the best predictor of diabetes remission for 1 year.[12]

4. There have been several early intensive therapy trials that have shown success in managing diabetes. Some effective strategies for people NEWLY diagnosed with type 2 diabetes include a very-low-calorie (800 kcal/daily) diet,[13,14] triple med therapy,[15] intensive insulin therapy,[16-23] and metabolic surgery.[24,25]

Case Summary and Closing Points

Type 2 diabetes is a chronic and progressive lifelong disease that is largely managed by the patient. Early treatment provides a long-term legacy effect and the longer we wait to take any action the less likely that action will be effective. Too many people have suffered from the "treat to fail" plan. Alternatively, we want to instill confidence and optimism among patients, giving them the tools to manage their diabetes with timely targeted therapies.

References

1. American Association of Diabetes Educators. AADE 7 Self-Care Behaviors. Accessed December 28, 2022. https://www.diabeteseducator.org/patient-resources/aade7-self-care-behaviors
2. Shubrook JH, Brannan GD, Klein G, Wapner A, Schwartz FL. Time needed for diabetes self-care: nationwide survey of certified diabetes educators. *Diabetes Spectr.* 2018;31(3):267-271. doi:10.2337/ds17-0077
3. ADA 2022 Pharmacologic Approach to Type 2 Diabetes (American Diabetes Association. Standards of Medical Care 2022. Pharmacologic Approach to Glycemic Control. 2022. https://diabetesjournals.org/care/article/45/Supplement_1/S125/138908/9-Pharmacologic-Approaches-to-Glycemic-Treatment
4. McGuire BE, Morrison TG, Hermanns N, et al. Short-form measures of diabetes-related emotional distress: the problem areas in diabetes scale (PAID)-5 and PAID-1. *Diabetologia.* 2010;53(1):66-69. doi:10.1007/s00125-009-1559-5
5. Fisher L, Glasgow RE, Mullan JT, Skaff MM, Polonsky WH. Development of a brief diabetes distress screening instrument. *Ann Fam Med.* 2008;6(3):246-252. doi:10.1370/afm.842
6. Kroenke K, Spitzer RL, Williams JBW. The Patient Health Questionnaire-2: validity of a two-item depression screener. *Med Care.* 2003;41(11):1284-1292. doi:10.1097/01.MLR.0000093487.78664.3C
7. Brown JB, Conner C, Nichols GA. Secondary failure of metformin monotherapy in clinical practice. *Diabetes Care.* 2010;33(3):501-506. doi:10.2337/dc09-1749
8. Gerich JE. Oral hypoglycemic agents. *N Engl J Med.* 1989;321(18):1231-1245. [Published erratum appears in *N Engl J Med.* 1990;322:71].
9. Moradi S, Sahebi Z, Ebrahim Valojerdi A, Rohani F, Ebrahimi H. The association between the number of office visits and the control of cardiovascular risk factors in Iranian patients with type 2 diabetes. *PLoS One.* 2017;12(6):e0179190.
10. Defronzo RA. Banting lecture. From the triumvirate to the ominous octet: a new paradigm for the treatment of type 2 diabetes mellitus. *Diabetes.* 2009;58(4):773-795. doi:10.2337/db09-9028
11. Kramer CK, Zinman B, Retnakaran R. Short term intensive insulin therapy in type 2 diabetes mellitus: a systematic review and meta-analysis. *Lancet Diabetes Endocrinol.* 2013;1:28-34.
12. Kramer CK, Zinman B, Choi H, Retnakaran R. Predictors of sustained drug free diabetes remission over 48 weeks following short term intensive insulin therapy in early type 2 diabetes. *BMJ Open Diabetes Res Care.* 2016;4(1):e000270.
13. Lean ME, Leslie WS, Barnes AC, et al. Primary care-led weight management for remission of type 2 diabetes (DiRECT): an open-label, cluster-randomised trial. *Lancet.* 2018;391(10120):541-551. doi:10.1016/S0140-6736(17)33102-1
14. Al-Mrabeh A, Hollingsworth KG, Shaw JAM, et al. 2-year remission of type 2 diabetes and pancreas morphology: a post-hoc analysis of the DiRECT open-label, cluster-randomised trial. *Lancet Diabetes Endocrinol.* 2020;8(12):939-948. Erratum in: Lancet Diabetes Endocrinol. 2020;8(12):e7.. doi: 10.1016/S2213-8587(20)30303-X
15. Abdul-Ghani MA, Puckett C, Triplitt C, et al. Initial combination therapy with metformin, pioglitazone and exenatide is more effective than sequential add-on therapy in subjects with new-onset

diabetes. Results from the Efficacy and Durability of Initial Combination Therapy for Type 2 Diabetes (EDICT): a randomized trial. *Diabetes Obes Metab.* 2015;17(3):268-275. doi: 10.1111/dom.12417

16. Retnakaran R, Choi H, Ye C, Kramer CK, Zinman B. Two-year trial of intermittent insulin therapy vs metformin for the preservation of β-cell function after initial short-term intensive insulin induction in early type 2 diabetes. *Diabetes Obes Metab.* 2018;20(6):1399-1407. doi: 10.1111/dom.13236

17. Ryan EA, Imes S, Wallace C. Short-term intensive insulin therapy in newly diagnosed type 2 diabetes. *Diabetes Care.* 2004;27(5):1028-1032.

18. Chandra ST, Priya G, Khurana ML, et al. Comparison of gliclazide with insulin as initial treatment modality in newly diagnosed type 2 diabetes. *Diabetes Technol Therapeut.* 2008;10(5):363-368.

19. Weng J, Li Y, XU W, et al. Effect of intensive insulin therapy on beta-cell function and glycaemic control in patients with newly diagnosed type 2 diabetes: a multicentre randomised parallel-group trial. *Lancet.* 2008;371(9626):1753-1760.

20. Li Y, Xu W, Liao Z, et al. Induction of long-term glycemic control in newly diagnosed type 2 diabetic patients is associated with improvement of beta-cell function.. *Diabetes Care.* 2004;27(11):2597-2602.

21. Hu Y, Li L, Xu Y, et al. Short-term intensive therapy in newly diagnosed type 2 diabetes partially restores both insulin sensitivity and beta cell function in subjects with long-term remission. *Diabetes Care.* 2011;34(8):1848-1853.

22. Shubrook JH, Jones SA. Basal-bolus analogue insulin therapy as initial treatment of type 2 diabetes mellitus: a case series. *Insulin.* 2010;5:100-105.

23. Presswala L, Shubrook JH. Intensive insulin therapy as the primary treatment of type 2 diabetes. *Clin Diabetes.* 2011;29(4):151-153.

24. Sheng B, Truong K, Spitler H, Zhang L, Tong X, Chen L. The long-term effects of bariatric surgery on type 2 diabetes remission, microvascular and macrovascular complications, and mortality: a systematic review and meta-analysis. *Obes Surg.* 2017;27(10):2724-2732. doi: 10.1007/s11695-017-2866-4

25. Mingrone G, Panunzi S, De Gaetano A, et al. Metabolic surgery versus conventional medical therapy in patients with type 2 diabetes: 10-year follow-up of an open-label, single-centre, randomised controlled trial. *Lancet.* 2021;397(10271):293-304. doi:10.1016/S0140-6736(20)32649-0

Case 2. Type 2 Adolescent

"Time is not our friend."

Let us return to the child in Chapter 1, Case 2.

A 14-year-old African American boy presents (with his parents) with concerns about a rash. The rash is present on the posterior neck. They are not sure how long it has been present. However, his teacher called with concerns about hygiene.

Medications: none

Allergies: none (medication, latex, food)

Family Medical History: type 2 diabetes in mom, maternal grandmother (MGM), and paternal grandmother; asthma in dad and brother.

Social History: lives at home with parents and younger sister. Currently in ninth grade. Doing only ok at school. Has socially withdrawn this year. No tobacco, alcohol, or recreational drugs. Eats school-supported breakfast and lunch. No regular physical activity. Enjoys online video games.

The family's goal for today's visit is to get rid of this rash.

Physical Exam: Ht. 5′6″, Wt. 293 lb, BMI 47.3, T 98.6, P 88, R 15, BP 138/80

HEENT: velvety rash along posterior neck and axilla—acanthosis nigricans

CV: normal

Resp: normal

Skin: pink stretch marks noted on the abdomen and shoulders
Truncal obesity

Other Lab Values:

Other Labs	Value	Reference Range
HbA1c	8.8%	<5.7% (normal)
TSH (thyroid-stimulating hormone)/free T4	0.48/1.42	0.4-4.5 mIU/L/0.8-1.8 µg/dL
UACr	376 mg/g	<30 mg/g

We confirmed that he had diabetes in Chapter 1, Case 2 and there is strong evidence that he has type 2 diabetes. If you are not convinced by the clinical presentation that he has type 2 diabetes, you certainly could order a C-peptide in combination with a glucose. His glucose was 144 mg/dL and the C-peptide is normal to high, which further supports the diagnosis of type 2 diabetes. Some health care professionals might order autoantibodies for this patient. While it is reasonable in any child diagnosed with diabetes, there is a low likelihood of being autoantibodies positive. There is also the possibility of a false positive result. For this reason, I would caution against this approach.

 CASE QUESTIONS

1. What are the treatment options for children with type 2 diabetes?
2. Is there a difference in treating children versus adults when it comes to type 2 diabetes?
3. What is the future of treating type 2 diabetes in children and adolescents?

 ANSWERS AND EXPLANATIONS

1. Type 2 diabetes in children is even more progressive than it is in adults.[1,2] Children and young adults who are diagnosed with T2DM have shorter periods before they start developing complications.[3,4] Therefore, treating type 2 diabetes aggressively and in a timely manner in children is very important.

   However, treating children who have metabolic disorders and who are overweight or obese is complicated. Most children work very hard just to "fit in." To be successful with this child, we will need to take a collaborative, family-focused approach. Children with metabolic conditions often struggle with shame and guilt. As a result, it is very important that lifestyle interventions focus on the entire family unit, to avoid isolating the child. Providing dietary education to create a healthy meal plan the entire family can benefit from should be a central focus.

   There is a clearly established link between food insecurity and the development of type 2 diabetes. Our patient is currently dependent on school-supported meals twice a day. He and his family may benefit from the assistance of a social worker to help identify food assistance resources.

If available, specialty centers that provide a multidisciplinary approach to the treatment of overweight or obese adolescents with type 2 diabetes often provide the best long-term health outcomes.[5] If a specialty center is not available, scheduling family appointments, and including a diabetes educator and dietician can help promote critical behavior changes.

2. Treating children with type 2 diabetes provides some unique challenges. While there are many treatment options for adults with type 2 diabetes, the choices are more limited for children and adolescents. Unfortunately, very few medications have been studied in children.[6] The most widely used therapies for children with type 2 diabetes include metformin and insulin. SUs are also used but only glimepiride has an indication in children aged 8 years and older. However, two GLP-1RAs have recently been approved for children aged 10 years and above.[7,8] Table 2.2 shows the Food and Drug Administration–approved treatments in children.[9]

Adherence to any treatment program for a chronic disease is hard for children. Starting with focused interdisciplinary approach may be the best option to help the child and family manage this condition. It may also allow for a reduction in medication in the future. This could provide positive feedback for the child and family and may also build confidence in the family's ability to use lifestyle measures to maintain control.

TABLE 2.2 Food and Drug Administration–Approved Diabetes Treatments for Children

Medication Class	Drugs	Minimum Age for Use
Biguanides	Metformin	10 years
SU	Glimepiride	8 years
Glucagon-like peptide-1 receptor agonist	Liraglutide	10 years
	Exenatide weekly	10 years
	Dulaglutide	10+ years
Insulins: basal	Glargine	6 years
	Detemir	2 years
	Degludec	1 year
Insulin: bolus/prandial	Insulin NPH	Not specified
	Insulin (R)	2 Years
	Insulin aspart	2 Years
	Insulin lispro	3 years
	Insulin glulisine	4 years

Sources: Peters A, Laffel L, et al; American Diabetes Association Transitions Working Group. Diabetes care for emerging adults: recommendations for transition from pediatric to adult diabetes care systems – a position statement of the American Diabetes Association, with representation by the American College of Osteopathic Family Physicians, the American Academy of Pediatrics, the American Association of Clinical Endocrinologists, the American Osteopathic Association, the Centers for Disease Control and Prevention, Children with Diabetes, The Endocrine Society, the International Society for Pediatric and Adolescent Diabetes, Juvenile Diabetes Research Foundation International, the National Diabetes Education Program, and the Pediatric Endocrine Society (formerly Lawson Wilkins Pediatric Endocrine Society). Molinari AM, Shubrook JH. Treatment options and current guidelines of care for pediatric type 2 diabetes patients: a narrative review. *J Osteopath Med.* 2021;121(4):431-440. doi:10.1515/jom-2020-0172. PMID: 33694353.

Second, treating children and adolescents requires both the patient and their guardian/parent to understand and consent to starting pharmacotherapy. Finally, we have to assume that all children with type 2 diabetes are of reproductive age so we will need to include this consideration when selecting a treatment option as even metformin has been reported to be tied to birth defects in offspring of men taking metformin.[10]

3. As we have come to appreciate the significance and severity of type 2 diabetes in children, we have recognized the importance of developing innovative approaches to treatment. Some centers have had success with metabolic surgery—to address the excess weight and metabolic abnormalities.[11] Newer medications such as SGLT-2 inhibitors, additional GLP-1RAs and the anticipated GLP-1/GIP combined agonists may have a role in the treatment of pediatric type 2 diabetes.[12]

While it was not a focus on this case, this patient also had albuminuria—or increased albumin excretion in the urine. This is an important finding and may be the first indication of a diabetes-related complication, specifically diabetes-related kidney disease.

Case Summary and Closing Points

Type 2 diabetes in younger people and adolescents is becoming more common. While this condition in younger people is more severe and more progressive, both health care professionals and families are generally more tentative when it comes to treatment. It is critical that clinicians communicate the severity of this condition and the importance of getting ahead of the disease instead of waiting and responding to inevitable complications. The bottom line, any delay may substantially affect the person's quality and quantity of life.

References

1. Dart AB, Martens PJ, Rigatto C, Brownell MD, Dean HJ, Sellers EA. Earlier onset of complications in youth with type 2 diabetes. *Diabetes Care*. 2014;37:436-443.
2. TODAY Study Group; Zeitler P, Epstein L, Grey M, et al. Treatment options for type 2 diabetes in adolescents and youth: a study of the comparative efficacy of metformin alone or in combination with rosiglitazone or lifestyle intervention in adolescents with type 2 diabetes. *Pediatr Diabetes*. 2007;8(2):74-87.
3. TODAY Study Group; Shah RD, Braffett BH, Tryggestad JB, et al. Cardiovascular risk factor progression in adolescents and young adults with youth-onset type 2 diabetes. *J Diabetes Complications*. 2022;36(3):108123. doi: 10.1016/j.jdiacomp.2021.108123
4. RISE Consortium. Lack of durable improvements in β-cell function following withdrawal of pharmacological interventions in adults with impaired glucose tolerance or recently diagnosed type 2 diabetes. *Diabetes Care*. 2019;42(9):1742-1751. doi:10.2337/dc19-0556
5. Seligman HK, Bindman AB, Vittinghoff E, Kanaya AM, Kushel MB. Food insecurity is associated with diabetes mellitus: results from the National Health Examination and Nutrition Examination Survey (NHANES) 1999-2002. *J Gen Intern Med*. 2007;22(7):1018-1023. doi: 10.1007/s11606-007-0192-6
6. Molinari AM, Shubrook JH. Treatment options and current guidelines of care for pediatric type 2 diabetes patients: a narrative review. *J Osteopath Med*. 2021;121(4):431-440. doi: 10.1515/jom-2020-0172
7. Package Insert Victoza. https://www.accessdata.fda.gov/drugsatfda_docs/label/2010/022341lbl.pdf
8. Package insert Bydureon Bcise. https://www.accessdata.fda.gov/drugsatfda_docs/label/2017/209210s000lbl.pdf
9. Peters A, Laffel L, et al; American Diabetes Association Transitions Working Group. Diabetes care for emerging adults: recommendations for transition from pediatric to adult diabetes care systems—a position statement of the American diabetes association, with representation by the American college of

osteopathic family physicians, the American Academy of pediatrics, the American association of clinical Endocrinologists, the American osteopathic association, the centers for disease control and prevention, children with diabetes, the Endocrine society, the international society for pediatric and adolescent diabetes, Juvenile diabetes Research Foundation international, the National diabetes education program, and the pediatric Endocrine society (formerly Lawson Wilkins pediatric Endocrine society). *Diabetes Care.* 2011;34(11):2477-2485. Erratum in: Diabetes Care. 2012;35(1):191. doi:10.2337/dc11-1723

10. Wensink MJ, Shaw GM, Lu Y, et al. Preconception antidiabetic drugs in men and birth defects in offspring: a Nationwide cohort study. *Ann Intern Med.* 2022;175(5):665-673. doi: 10.7326/M21-4389
11. Till H, Mann O, Singer G, Weihrauch-Blüher S. Update on metabolic bariatric surgery for morbidly obese adolescents. *Children (Basel).* 2021;8(5):372. doi: 10.3390/children8050372
12. ClinicalTrialsgov. A Study to Evaluate Tirzepatide (LY3298176) in Pediatric and Adolescent Participants With Type 2 Diabetes Mellitus Inadequately Controlled With Metformin or Basal Insulin or Both (SURPASS-PEDS). Accessed December 28, 2022. https://clinicaltrials.gov/ct2/show/NCT05260021

Case 3. Type 1 Child

"This is not going away."

Return to the child in Chapter 1, Case 3. He was diagnosed with type 1 diabetes when he was admitted to the hospital with diabetic ketoacidosis (DKA). This is a summary of his initial presentation: An 8-year-old boy presents to the emergency room (ER) with a stomach flu that does not seem to be resolving. His mom explains that he started acting differently a couple of weeks ago. He came home from a sleepover, and she noticed that he was drinking a lot and peeing a lot. He also seemed to be more hungry than normal. This has persisted for several weeks. Also, his mom noticed that he was losing weight. While changes in eating were common for him with growth spurts, weight loss was not. In the last 2 days things have worsened, as he has abdominal pain, nausea, and has vomited several times.

Medications: none

Allergies: none

Family Medical History: immediate family in good health, Alzheimer disease in MGM

Social History: lives with his parents, one older sister, and one younger brother; normal developmental milestones; "picky" eater; doing well in school, fourth grade

Physical Exam

Vitals: HR 98, R 26, T 98.6 °F, BP 98/68, Ht. 52 in, Wt. 70 lb, BMI 18.2

General: alert and responsive

HEENT: normal

Heart: regular rate and rhythm

Lungs: tachypneic, clear in anterior and posterior fields

Abdomen: BS (bowel sounds) active, benign

It has been 6 weeks since that hospitalization. He is feeling more comfortable checking his glucose (which he can do alone) and he is able to give his injections but needs help calculating his insulin dose. He is currently taking insulin glargine 12 units each morning and insulin aspart 4 units before each meal. He takes his glargine in his buttocks and he injects aspart in his arms and thighs. He is nervous about injecting in his abdomen. He used to snack a lot but has been trying to pay more attention to his diet.

His family has noticed he seems to be needing less insulin and sometimes his blood sugar drops too low. They get very scared when this happens. The father is wondering if his diabetes is "getting better" and if he will not need insulin after all. He mentions that his son really does not like taking his injections. He and his mother hope at some point he will no longer need to use insulin.

The parents also want to know if this is something their other children are going to get and what is the "real cause" of his diabetes?

 ## CASE QUESTIONS

1. Why is he needing less insulin?
2. What do you recommend about injection sites?
3. What do you recommend about snacking and nutrition?
4. How can we help him become more comfortable with insulin injections?
5. How would you address the family question about the "real cause" of diabetes and the risk for siblings to develop type 1 diabetes?

 ## ANSWERS AND EXPLANATIONS

1. Many people with type 1 diabetes will experience a temporary "rebound" in pancreatic beta cell function once exogenous insulin is started. This is commonly termed the "honeymoon period." It is very important for the patient and family to understand that while he may need less insulin during the honeymoon period, the improvement will not be permanent; his diabetes is not going away nor is it "cured."[1,2]

   The "honeymoon period" typically has a mean duration of about 3 months; on rare occasions it may last more than 1 year. During the honeymoon phase pancreatic beta cell function improves enough that one's insulin requirements are significantly decreased. Rarely, exogenous insulin may not be needed at all.

   This is a great time to highlight to the family that with exogenous insulin administration the demands on the beta cells are reduced. As a result, this may reduce the body's autoimmune attack on the pancreas. Any residual beta cell secretion may be temporarily spared. Beta cell function preserved for a short period of time, yielding even a small amount of insulin production, can be helpful for the long-term management of this patient's diabetes. This scenario is termed "micro-secretion." Patients who are micro-secretors often have longer periods of time before complications occur and can have a lower risk of severe glucose excursions and sometimes a lower risk of microvascular complications.[3]

   Due to the complex nature of type 1 diabetes disease management, affected children and their families often require a great deal of support. It is recommended that this care be provided in specialty diabetes centers with access to diabetes educators, dietitians, and social support.[4,5]

2. As of 2022, people with type 1 diabetes will need to use subcutaneous insulin for their entire life. Currently all but one type of insulin is administered by subcutaneous injection. Typically, people with type 1 diabetes will require 3 to 8 insulin injections per day.

   It is important for people who inject insulin to use multiple injection sites. It is best to inject into an area of fatty tissue and to avoid injecting directly over muscle, as insulin injected over muscle tissue may be absorbed more rapidly. For many people the abdomen is the injection site that provides the most reliable absorption of insulin. I often recommend starting injections in the abdomen and not introducing other sites until the person is comfortable with the abdomen as an injection site. Patients may need reassurance that performing abdominal injection is safe. They also may be fearful that abdominal injection will be more painful than injections elsewhere. Injection sites should be rotated on a regular basis to prevent the development of lipohypertrophy and/or subcutaneous scar tissue formation, both of which may interfere with insulin absorption. Newly diagnosed patients should be trained at administering their insulin at different injection sites and practice doing so. Once they are comfortable with their options, the patient can decide where to inject based upon individual preference and convenience.[6] Potential injection sites can be seen in Figure 2.1.

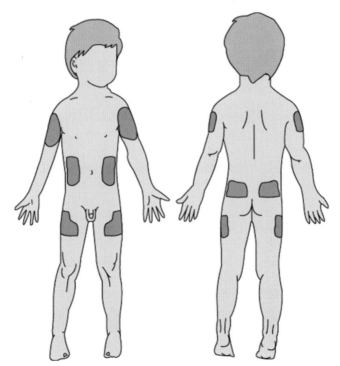

FIGURE 2.1. Potential injection sites. According to the American Diabetes Association, insulin injection sites in children and adults are the upper outer portions of the arms; the thighs, 4 in. below the hip and 4 in. above the knee (adjusted proportionally for children); and the abdominal area just above and just below the waist. The navel and a circular area just around it are excluded as injection sites. In some children, the abdominal area may not be an appropriate injection site. (Used with permission from Silbert-Flagg J. *Maternal & Child Health Nursing*. 9th ed. Wolters Kluwer. 2022.)

3. Learning how to successfully manage mealtime insulin dosing can be challenging. Early on it may be best for the person to decide what meals they like the most and focus on developing carbohydrate consistency as they learn about their prandial insulin requirements. This is one of the earliest steps in understanding the relationship between carbohydrate ingestion and insulin needed to maintain glycemic control. Once they learn the nutrition content of their meals and the insulin requirement it can help to guide a "carbohydrate count."

   Carb counting is used to help people take a certain amount of insulin to match a certain amount of carbs in a meal. While carb counting is a challenging skill to learn, there are many helpful tools available to make the process easier. Numerous phone applications such as MyFitnessPal, CalorieKing, Lose It, Glucose Buddy, and others are available to help estimate the carb content of many fast foods as well as foods prepared at home.

   The same concept of carb counting applies to snacking. Once a person realizes that there is a balance between carbohydrates ingested and insulin administered, the person may start to modify both sides of the equation. This is normal and expected. Just as with people without diabetes, excessive snacking may lead to undesired weight gain. Not uncommonly patients may develop a distorted view of their relationship with food, and their insulin requirements. Some people will take it to an extreme and try to avoid carbohydrates to avoid needing to take insulin. This can become maladaptive over time, and often leads to poor glycemic control.

   Disordered eating is very common in type 1 diabetes.[7] Young women with DM1 are twice as likely as people without diabetes to have an eating disorder.[7] Diabulimia or insulin purging is the second most common method of weight loss (behind dieting) among this population.[7] It is often associated with poorer regimen adherence, poor glycemic control, and higher rates of complications. Because there is a direct association between one's dietary habits and their diabetes management, every effort should be made to help the person maintain a healthy relationship with food. Patients should be reassured that they need not lose their joy of eating (Table 2.3).

4. For many patients the thought of giving themselves injections can be overwhelming. Patients with type 1 diabetes typically receive specific training on injection technique at the time of diagnosis. This is not always the case with patients with type 2 diabetes. If a person is reluctant to take injections, it is worth exploring what

TABLE 2.3 Applications to Assist With Carb Counting and Glucose Management			
Apps for Carb Content/Nutrition Facts		Apps to Assist With Glucose Tracking and Review	Apps to Assist With Insulin Dosing
MyFitnessPal	MyNetDiary	mySugr	RapidCalc
CalorieKing	Carb Manager	OneDrop	
Lose It	Fooducate	Glucose Buddy	
Glucose Buddy		Glooko	

their main challenges are. Is it the idea of injection itself, apprehension of pain, the length of the needle, fear of misdosing, or lack of confidence in their injection technique? Learning more about their perceived barriers can help you problem-solve together, and develop a solution for the patient.

Often it can simply be the inconvenience of needing to administer insulin in a public setting, and the need to carry their insulin with them. Historically, many people were prescribed insulin vials and syringes. While this may be an efficient way to administer insulin, it can be cumbersome to give doses outside of the home. Vials need to be maintained at temperatures between 36 and 46 °F. Hence, one would need to carry their insulin with them in a refrigerated bag or cooler.

Many people prefer to use insulin pens. These can be carried without refrigeration (2-5 weeks depending on the insulin). They are preloaded, so patients do not have to worry about drawing the insulin into a syringe. For many people it is easier to dial in their insulin dose on a pen, than to visualize it on a syringe. Because the pen is reusable, patients do not need to worry about disposing of used syringes, or the amount of paraphernalia they must carry with them.

For those patients lacking confidence in their injection technique, there are devices that help show them where to inject and even one that creates an injection site for them, so they do not need to worry about breaking the skin when they are injecting away from home.

Patients may become frustrated with the need to perform multiple daily insulin injections and frequent fingerstick glucose monitoring. There are tools available to reduce the burden of these tasks and can even make dosing more specific and safer. Continuous glucose monitors can assist in providing ongoing glucose levels without the need for fingersticks. Most systems do not require glucose calibration and are compatible with smartphones to allow people to use their phone to see current glucose readings, follow trends, and even provide alerts for high or low glucose levels. Providers are also able to acquire data remotely.

Insulin pumps provide a refined way to replace injections for insulin delivery. These are attractive for many people with type 1 diabetes as they can replace basal, mealtime, and correction insulin doses. Insulin pumps provide a continuous subcutaneous infusion of rapid acting insulin to meet basal insulin needs, as well as mealtime and correction needs by bolus delivery from the same system. We will discuss these devices in Chapter 7.

5. Receiving a new diagnosis of type 1 diabetes is often traumatic and overwhelming for the patient and their family. It is very common for them to come back weeks, months, or even years later to ask about why this happened, and how it could have been prevented. It is very important to provide up-to-date medical knowledge about their disease at a level the patient can understand, and to identify areas where there are still knowledge gaps.

For example, it is important to share that the development of type 1 diabetes is a result of a complex combination of specific genetic markers (often spontaneous mutations) combined with common environmental triggers that do little harm in most people, but in people with genetic risk, can activate an abnormal immune response.

TABLE 2.4   Risk of Developing Type 1 Diabetes Based on the Family Member With Type 1 Diabetes Mellitus (T1DM)

	T1 Diabetes Risk
General population	0.4%
Father w/ T1DM	4%-7%
Mother with T1DM	1.5%-3%
Sibling with T1DM	6%-7%
Identical twin with T1DM	30%-70%

From Parkkola A, Härkönen T, Ryhänen SJ, Ilonen J, Knip M; Finnish Pediatric Diabetes Register. Extended family history of type 1 diabetes and phenotype and genotype of newly diagnosed children. *Diabetes Care*. 2013;36(2):348-354. doi:10.2337/dc12 to 0445. Epub October 1, 2012. Turtinen M, Härkönen T, Parkkola A, Ilonen J, Knip M; Finnish Pediatric Diabetes Register. Characteristics of familial type 1 diabetes: effects of the relationship to the affected family member on phenotype and genotype at diagnosis. *Diabetologia*. 2019;62(11):2025 to 2039. doi:10.1007/s00125-019-4952-8.

Many families want to know about the risk of type 1 diabetes for other family members. While type 2 diabetes can be an inherited condition, the same is not true for most people with type 1 diabetes. More than 93% of people with type 1 diabetes have no family history.[8] However, as seen in Table 2.4 there is a small increase in prevalence if a close relative has type 1 diabetes mellitus (T1DM).[9]

Case Summary and Closing Points

A new diagnosis of type 1 is a life changing event for all involved. More so than with any other form of diabetes, a hospital admission and intensive education can really help the family to start the learning process effectively and adjust successfully. That being said, learning to live with diabetes will be an ongoing endeavor, and each new situation may be a learning opportunity. Close and frequent contact among the patient, clinician, and family is a critical ingredient for success aka a higher quality of life.

References

1. Sokołowska M, Chobot A, Jarosz-Chobot P. The honeymoon phase - what we know today about the factors that can modulate the remission period in type 1 diabetes. *Pediatr Endocrinol Diabetes Metab*. 2016;22(2):66-70. English. doi:10.18544/PEDM-22.02.0053
2. Abdul-Rasoul M, Habib H, Al-Khouly M. The honeymoon phase' in children with type 1 diabetes mellitus: frequency, duration, and influential factors. *Pediatr Diabetes*. 2006;7(2):101-107. doi:10.1111/j.1399-543X.2006.00155.x
3. Keenan HA, Sun JK, Levine J, et al. Residual insulin production and pancreatic ß-cell turnover after 50 years of diabetes: Joslin Medalist Study. *Diabetes*. 2010;59(11):2846-2853. doi:10.2337/db10-0676
4. Sperling MA, Laffel LM. Current management of glycemia in children with type 1 diabetes mellitus. *N Engl J Med*. 2022;386(12):1155-1164. doi:10.1056/NEJMcp2112175
5. Chiang JL, Maahs DM, Garvey KC, et al. Type 1 diabetes in children and adolescents: a position statement by the American diabetes association. *Diabetes Care*. 2018;41(9):2026-2044. doi:10.2337/dci18-0023
6. Silbert-Flagg J. *Maternal & Child Health Nursing*. 9th ed. Wolters Kluwer. 2022.

7. Hanlan ME, Griffith J, Patel N, Jaser SS. Eating disorders and disordered eating in type 1 diabetes: prevalence, screening, and treatment options. *Curr Diab Rep*. Published online 2013. doi:10.1007/s11892-013-0418-4

8. Parkkola A, Härkönen T, Ryhänen SJ, Ilonen J, Knip M; Finnish Pediatric Diabetes Register. Extended family history of type 1 diabetes and phenotype and genotype of newly diagnosed children. *Diabetes Care*. 2013;36(2):348-354. doi:10.2337/dc12-0445

9. Turtinen M, Härkönen T, Parkkola A, Ilonen J, Knip M; Finnish Pediatric Diabetes Register. Characteristics of familial type 1 diabetes: effects of the relationship to the affected family member on phenotype and genotype at diagnosis. *Diabetologia*. 2019;62(11):2025-2039. doi:10.1007/s00125-019-4952-8

Case 4. Type 1 Young Adulthood

"We can make it a bit easier living with type 1."

A 26-year-old man presents to you to establish care. He has type 1 diabetes, which was first diagnosed when he was 14 years old. He remembers this specifically because he was admitted to his local hospital's ICU in DKA on his 14th birthday. His initial care was at the Children's Hospital Diabetes Center closest to his home. During college he would return periodically to this center for his care. He recently moved further from his home to start graduate school and would like to have a local health care provider who can help him manage his diabetes.

He has always had a hard time controlling his diabetes. During college he did not devote much effort to regulating his diet and managing his blood sugar. He knows he needs to pay more attention to this. He lives with two roommates who are aware he has diabetes, but do not really understand what this means and what he needs to do to take care of himself. Being new to the area, he has not met anyone else who has diabetes. He generally does not share that he has diabetes with many people. He has specifically avoided discussing this with former girlfriends because "it made things complicated."

He was referred to you after being seen in the ER last week. He went there because his blood sugar was climbing, and he did not want to go into DKA again. He recently aged out of his parent's insurance and ran out of insulin. He has been using insulin detemir by vial 38 units each morning and estimates his insulin lispro dose based on what he is eating. His lispro dose range is 2 to 6 units per meal. He typically injects in either his arms or his legs, but sometimes hits hard spots. His diet is not as good as it should be. He eats a lot of fast food, and often will eat whatever his roommates are having. He checks his blood sugars when he can, but knows he is not testing as often as he should because of his busy schedule. He has occasional lows, which he addresses with a cup of juice or soda. He used to have a glucagon pen for emergencies but does not have one anymore.

He says he needs all of his medications and supplies refilled.

Past Medical History: type 1 diabetes

Medications: insulin detemir, insulin lispro

Allergies: none

Family Medical History: hypothyroidism in mom

Social History: lives with 2 roommates. No tobacco, alcohol or recreational drug use

Physical Exam

Vitals: HR 72, R 12, T 98.6 °F, BP 108/74, Ht. 66 inches, Wt. 148 lb, BMI 23.89

General: alert and responsive

HEENT: normal

Heart: regular rate and rhythm

Lungs: clear in anterior and posterior fields

Abdomen: BS active, benign

Extremities: normal pulses, no skin changes, monofilament exam is normal bilaterally.

 ## CASE QUESTIONS

1. What are the challenges that need to be addressed?
2. What constitutes "all of his medications and supplies"?
3. What advice would you provide in terms of diabetes treatment?

 ## ANSWERS AND EXPLANATIONS

1. Most children entering adulthood with type 1 diabetes will have been treated in pediatric diabetes specialty centers. This care typically starts at the time of diagnosis and continues until age 18 to 25 years but may continue well into adulthood. Pediatric diabetes specialty care is much different than most adult care in the United States. When patients "age out" of their pediatric care, they often find it challenging to adjust to the adult care system. The ADA provided a multiple specialty consensus statement to assist in the care of the emerging adult with diabetes.[1]

   Most young adults have not been responsible for obtaining their medications and supplies. Often the diabetes education they received at diagnosis was relevant for a child, but not for an independent adult. As they transition into adulthood and assume the primary role of managing their care, their educational needs will change.

   Previously, their treatment options were largely decided by their parents or guardians. Young adults may become overwhelmed when health care professionals ask their preferences for care or suggest regimens different from what they are accustomed to. Our patient may know what "works" for him, but his definition of "working" may be the prevention of severe hypoglycemia, or hyperglycemia requiring emergency care.

   At this initial visit with a young adult, I think there are some very fundamental things we can do to help. First, it is important to take the time to hear about their diabetes experience. I often ask them to tell me about their "diabetes story." Most people with type 1 diabetes remember the exact day their diabetes was diagnosed. This shows the impact the diagnosis may have had in their life.

Then I like to ask what their goals are for the visit. This is important; giving the patient a voice early in the relationship will help them to see that you are interested and can be an ally in their care.

Next, I share with my patients that I understand living with type 1 diabetes can be hard. I will work with them to provide guidance, support, and technology to help make it a bit easier to manage. I let them know this will be a partnership. I offer suggestions and options, but I make it clear that they will need to let me know what will work for them, since diabetes is largely self-managed.

The other thing to establish is "who is on their diabetes team"? These are the people who know they have diabetes and can provide support when needed. Often, young people with diabetes do not share with people around them that they have diabetes. This patient needs people around him who can help if he is going high or low and aid with treatment if needed. It is also helpful for people with type 1 diabetes to know other people with type 1 diabetes. Developing a peer group is a good way to address the sense of isolation people with diabetes may experience. It is also a great way to share "tricks of the trade" and learn about available resources in their community.

For today, our patient needs all his medication and supplies refilled. I encourage patients with T1DM to have a checklist of their medications and supplies available at each visit. We will address this more in the next question.

    Key topics to address with the emerging adult with diabetes:
- Concern about injection sites
- Medical home for his care
- Discussion of glucagon, ketone strips
- Repeat diabetes education as an adult
- Discuss support system and being transparent
- Introduce technology

2. While this may seem straightforward, it is critical that we get all of the needed supplies to our patients with type 1 diabetes. I recommend that you have a set checklist that the patients can help fill out to make sure we get everything they need (Table 2.5).

    The ADA has a great website resource to help identify all of the diabetes-related supplies. This is also found in Spring Issue of *Diabetes Forecast*. To find diabetes educators, diabetes care providers, and online resources, you can visit the ADA Support page: https://www.diabetes.org/tools-support-.[2] To find all tolls as it relates to diabetes, you can visit the ADA Consumer guide page: https://consumerguide.diabetes.org/-.[3]

    Key items that patients with type 1 diabetes will need prescriptions for:
- Supplies for insulin
- Supplies for testing
- Glucagon, ketone strips, and sharps

3. At the initial visit our goal may be to establish a relationship and to provide the patient with their needed medications and supplies. Offering to be an ally and to

TABLE 2.5 Diabetes Supplies Checklist			
How Do You Take Your Insulin?	**Vial and Syringe**	**Insulin Pens**	**Insulin Pump**
What is your basal insulin and dose? What is your mealtime insulin?			(Basal rate)—do you have backup insulin if your pump fails?
How do you dose insulin at meals? Carb count/fixed amount/small meal large meal?	Carb count		
How do you correct a high glucose? Correction factor, correction scale?			
Testing Supplies			
What glucose meter do you have?			
Do you have a backup meter?			
What test strips do you use?			
How many times per day do you test your glucose?			
Do you have a lancing device?			
Do you have control solution?			
Emergency Supplies			
Do you have glucose tabs/rapid glucose source? Do you carry with you at all times?			
Do you have glucagon? Which formulation and how old is it?			
Do you have ketone strips—urine or blood? How old are they?			
Do you have an emergency diabetes ID? Bracelet, necklace, wallet insert, tattoo?			
Who is your emergency contact? Do they know your highs and lows? Do they know how to give glucagon?			

support their self-management via information and technology sends the message that we care and can be more than just a source for their prescriptions.

It is important to provide some guidance regarding anticipated frequency of visits, and a typical visit agenda. I like to share how they can access care during times of crisis or emergency, and any support services that are available. If the patient is interested in suggestions for treatment, we can discuss options. For this patient, providing prescriptions for insulin and necessary supplies will likely make a significant difference in their overall glucose control.

For many people their focus is on the control of hyperglycemia. They are less worried about hypoglycemia. It is important to discuss the dangers associated with hypoglycemia particularly if the patient is hypoglycemic unaware. Educating the patient on the recognition of hypoglycemia and appropriate management of hypoglycemic episodes can help them feel safer and reduce the incidence of rebound hyperglycemia.

Many people with type 1 diabetes are not fully aware of novel management options. As our patient is new to his insurance, he may not be familiar with coverage for technology items such as CGM systems and insulin pumps. This is a great time to share what some of his options are and how he can access them. I direct patients to a helpful website: https://diabeteswise.org/#/.[4] This site was developed by researchers from Stanford and provides people with diabetes information on the full spectrum of available diabetes technology. It also includes patient stories and even an initial quiz to help the person find out what might be good options for them. There is also a site for healthcare professionals who want to learn more about diabetes technology and devices. The site is https://pro.diabeteswise.org/#/.[5]

Advanced skills for the person with type 1 diabetes:

- Reengage carb counting as a way to free up lifestyle
- Handling glucose during special situations—exercise, alcohol, travel
- Discuss hypoglycemic unawareness
- Introduce technology and benefits of new insurance

Case Summary and Closing Points

The needs of an emerging adult with type 1 diabetes are unique. Recall that the organization and experience of pediatric care are substantially different than adult health care. The transition of responsibility from a caregiver to the patient themselves will vary. Assessing where an individual patient is at in the assumption of their own care will help the provider individualize information and messaging to greatest effect. Finally, most people with type 1 diabetes by this age have learned "what works for them" and may be resistant to changes as a general rule. The best approach is to get to know the patient first before making any major changes.

References

1. Peters A, Laffel L; American Diabetes Association Transitions Working Group. Diabetes care for emerging adults: recommendations for transition from pediatric to adult diabetes care systems—a position statement of the American diabetes association, with representation by the American college of osteopathic family physicians, the American Academy of pediatrics, the American association of clinical Endocrinologists, the American osteopathic association, the centers for disease control and prevention, children with diabetes, the Endocrine society, the international society for pediatric and adolescent diabetes, Juvenile diabetes Research Foundation international, the National diabetes education program, and the pediatric Endocrine society (formerly Lawson Wilkins pediatric Endocrine society). *Diabetes Care*. 2011;34(11):2477-2485. Erratum in: Diabetes Care. 2012;35(1):191. doi:10.2337/dc11-1723
2. ADA Support page. Accessed December 28, 2022. https://www.diabetes.org/tools-support
3. ADA Consumer guide. Accessed December 28, 2022. https://consumerguide.diabetes.org/
4. DiabetesWise website. Accessed December 28, 2022. https://diabeteswise.org/#/
5. DiabetesWise Pro website. Accessed December 28, 2022. https://pro.diabeteswise.org/#/

Case 5.   Developing an Engaged Family Approach

"We are all in this together."

A 44-year-old woman presents to go over recent annual labs. She has generally been feeling well but acknowledges that during the COVID-19 pandemic she was getting out in the world much less. As a result, she has been less active and has been snacking more. She suspects as a result, her cholesterol levels will be higher.

She has been living with her sister. She mentions it has been nice to be with someone during these challenging times, but her sister really likes to eat at night, and the nighttime movie marathons with snacks included have become pretty common.

Past Medical History: dyslipidemia, OA thumbs

Medications: pravastatin 20 mg daily

Allergies: none

Family Medical History: parents deceased: mom, type 2 diabetes and stroke; dad, MI; sister, obesity and high cholesterol

Social History: lives with her sister, eating has been more liberal and intake greater at night. Works as a school administrator but has been working from home for the last 2 years, no other regular physical activity. No tobacco, rare alcohol. Not sexually active.

Physical Exam

Vitals: HR 72, R 14, BP 136/82, Ht. 66 in, Wt. 204 lb, BMI 32.9

General: truncal obesity

CV: normal

Resp: normal

Psych: affect and mood normal

Exam otherwise normal

Labs Values:

Lipid Panel	Value	Reference Range
Cholesterol, total	248	125-200 mg/dL
Triglycerides	166	<150 mg/dL
LDL (calculated)	138	<130 mg/dL
HDL, cholesterol	40	>40 mg/dL men; >50 women
Non-HDL cholesterol	208	<130
Other Labs	**Value**	**Reference Range**
HbA1c	8.4%	<5.7% (normal)
UACr	48 mg/G	<30 mg/G
eGFR	98 mL/min	>60 mL/min/1.73 m^2

CASE QUESTIONS

1. What role the COVID-19 pandemic has on diabetes?
2. What type of diabetes does she have?
3. What can we do to help her manage her diabetes?

 ANSWERS AND EXPLANATIONS

1. Obesity is a major risk factor for type 2 diabetes mellitus. The 2017 to 2018 National Health and Nutrition Examination survey showed that approximately 82.6% of Americans have a BMI greater than 25 kg/m².[1] One in three US adults have prediabetes and 90% of those individuals are unaware of their condition,[2] and 20% of people with diabetes do not know that they have it.[2]

   One of the numerous consequences of the COVID-19 pandemic for many people was weight gain.[3] The stay-at-home orders and widespread closures of workplaces, gyms, parks, and entertainment venues left people with fewer options for physical activity.[4] As a consequence, a great deal of adults became more sedentary during the COVID-19 pandemic.[5] The COVID-19 at-home restrictions led to a greater than 28% increase in sedentary time.[6] As a result, the stay-at-home mandates were associated with weight gain in US adults, with the most weight gain in the obese baseline group.[4] With the many closures, the workforce also decreased during the COVID-19 pandemic. In the United States, unemployment reached its highest levels in April 2020, a month after the lockdowns began.[7] A pre-COVID-19-pandemic survey found that after 4 to 6 months of unemployment, people began increasing their consumption of sugars and carbohydrates.[8,9] Even health professionals saw a net increase in weight gain and decrease in physical activity during the COVID-19 pandemic.[10]

   Obesity, sedentary lifestyle, and high carbohydrate intake are all known risk factors for the development of T2DM.

   Recent literature has established that there may be an increase in the risk of both type 1 and type 2 diabetes after infection with COVID-19. A recent study found that in people who were infected with COVID-19 the subsequent risk of de novo diabetes increased by as much as 40%.[11]

2. This is a middle-aged adult who has a family history of type 2 diabetes and has risk factors for diabetes including dyslipidemia and obesity. She presented without specific symptoms suggestive of diabetes. Abnormal measures of glycemic control were found on screening lab testing. This is the most common presentation for type 2 diabetes. No further testing for other forms of diabetes is needed at this time.

3. This patient had significant lifestyle changes during the COVID-19 pandemic. However, she was already at increased risk for developing T2DM. Encouraging her to adopt a healthier lifestyle is fundamental. For most people, day-to-day decisions that impact our lives are not made in isolation. They are made within the context of our home, family, friends, and work environment. Addressing these interactions is vitally important to help people make successful lifestyle changes.

Primary care is well situated to help families manage and control diabetes. This requires insight into the patient's living circumstances and important relationships. If our patient attempts to make changes but her sister is still snacking at night, it will be much harder for our patient to succeed. Including this patient's sister in the lifestyle modification process can be critical in helping them both take steps toward better health. Recognizing that she is also at risk for developing diabetes may also help motivate our patient's sister to support her efforts. Having a visit with the patient and her sister can bring them together to work as a team to tackle diabetes.

It is also helpful to ask the patient to reflect on the other important people in her life, and encourage her to recruit them as partners for healthy lifestyle change.

Case Summary and Closing Points

While diabetes is often thought of as a condition that affects the individual, this is rarely the case. Diabetes mellitus is self-managed, but more often than not, making the necessary changes to manage diabetes effectively means including the efforts of family members and friends as well. Best practices, then, should include learning who the patient's key partners and influencers are and encouraging their active involvement toward helping the patient achieve their goals through healthy living and consistent adherence to a shared treatment plan.

References

1. Fryar CD, Carroll MD, Afful J. *Prevalence of Overweight, Obesity, and Severe Obesity Among Adults Aged 20 and over: United States, 1960-1962 through 2017-2018*; 2020. https://www.cdc.gov/nchs/data/hestat/obesity-adult-17-18/overweight-obesity-adults-H.pdf
2. *Diabetes and Prediabetes | CDC.* 2020. www.cdc.gov. https://www.cdc.gov/chronicdisease/resources/publications/factsheets/diabetes-prediabetes.htm#prediabetes
3. Seal A, Schaffner A, Phelan S, et al. COVID-19 pandemic and stay-at-home mandates promote weight gain in US adults. *Obesity.* 2022;30(1):240-248. doi:10.1002/oby.23293
4. Czeisler EM, Tynan AM, Howard EM, et al. Public attitudes, behaviors, and beliefs related to COVID-19, stay-at-home orders, Nonessential business closures, and public health guidance—United States, New York city, and los angeles, may 5-12, 2020. *CDC Morbidity and Mortality Weekly Report (MMWR).* 2020;69(24):751-758. Retrieved from May 5, 2021. doi:10.15585/mmwr.mm6924e1external icon
5. Flanagan EW, Beyl RA, Fearnbach SN, Altazan AD, Martin CK, Redman LM. The impact of COVID-19 stay-at-home orders on health behaviors in adults. *Obesity.* 2021;29(2):438-445. doi:10.1002/oby.23066
6. Ammar A, Brach M, Trabelsi K, et al. Effects of COVID-19 home confinement on eating behaviour and physical activity: results of the ECLB-COVID19 international online survey. *Nutrients.* 2020;12(6):1583. doi:10.3390/nu12061583
7. Falk G, Carter JA, Nicchitta IA, Nyhof EC, Romero PD. 2021. Unemployment Rates During the COVID-19 Pandemic: In Brief. *Congressional Research Service.* Retrieved from May 3, 2020 https://fas.org/sgp/crs/misc/R46554.pdf. https://fas.org/sgp/crs/misc/R46554.pdf
8. Smed S, Tetens I, Bøker Lund T, Holm L, Ljungdalh Nielsen A. The consequences of unemployment on diet composition and purchase behaviour: a longitudinal study from Denmark. *Public Health Nutr.* 2018;21(3):580-592. doi:10.1017/S136898001700266X
9. Drago L, Gonzalez A, Molitch M. Diabetes and nutrition: carbohydrates. *J Clin Endocrinol Metab.* 2008;93(3):E1. oi:10.1210/jcem.93.3.9994
10. Kiwan R, Unni E, Shubrook JH. *The Effects of COVID-19 Pandemic Lock Down on Body Weight and Risk Score for Diabetes among Healthcare Students.* Unpublished data.
11. Xie Y, Al-Aly Z. Risks and burdens of incident diabetes in long COVID: a Cohort Study. *Lancet Diabetes Endocrinol.* 2022;10(5):311-321. doi:10.1016/S2213-8587(22)00044-4

Key Aspects of Treatment

Introduction

Having a plan and taking action are key aspects of helping people manage their diabetes. It is also important to recognize that, because diabetes is a chronic lifelong condition, the needs of the patient and clinical support offered will need to change over time. This chapter focuses on key aspects of diabetes management at different points in the progression of diabetes. Early in diabetes a full-court press may be the best plan. However, in the chronic phase, building support is most important for people with diabetes. Finally, it is important to balance the risks and benefits of treatment, understanding that later in the disease, deintensification is prudent.

Case 1.   Type 2 Is Progressive

"How do I cure my diabetes?"

A 36-year-old man presents to discuss treatment recommendations for his newly diagnosed diabetes. He recently completed his physical for work and learned he had glucose in his urine. Subsequent blood tests revealed a fasting glucose of 164 mg/dL and an A1c of 8.2%. He is surprised by the diagnosis, because he has been feeling fine, and did not have any idea that something was wrong. However, in hindsight he recognized that he often felt very sleepy after meals.

Med HX: no chronic problems

Medications: occasional OTC (over-the-counter) ibuprofen for joint pain or back pain

Allergies: none

Family Medical History: obesity is present in all immediate family members; dad has high cholesterol

Social History: no tobacco, no alcohol, and no recreational drug use. He lives with his spouse and three kids; ages 8, 6, and 2. He works as an accountant and this winter and spring have been tough as he is doing a lot of tax preparation.

He has heard you can "reverse" diabetes and he is "all in" to do this. He just needs to know the plan. He has coworkers who have struggled with diabetes-related complications and wants to do anything he can to avoid being like them. He is open to doing whatever he has to, including "big changes" in lifestyle. He is willing to start medications but would prefer not to need them forever.

Physical Exam: Ht. 5′7″, Wt. 200 lb, BMI 31.3, T 98.2, P 92, R 12, BP 126/72

GEN: obese adult, in no distress

HEENT: normal including thyroid exam

CV: normal

RESP: normal

Otherwise: normal exam

CASE QUESTIONS

1. Can type 2 diabetes be "reversed"?
2. What is the best treatment plan for this patient?
3. Should he start on medications? If yes, which ones?
4. What is the strategy to get this patient off medications?

 ANSWERS AND EXPLANATIONS

1. This is an important question, and the wording is key. There are plenty of references in the lay literature of "reversing" or "curing" type 2 diabetes. Current thinking is that it takes years of metabolic abnormalities and compensatory physiologic responses before a person becomes hyperglycemic from type 2 diabetes. While it is attractive to seek out a quick fix to "cure" type 2 diabetes, the truth is that there is no quick fix. It is important to remember that there are many pathways in the body that are altered in response to insulin resistance and abnormal insulin and glucose levels.

   However, there are many studies that have demonstrated that type 2 diabetes can be put into remission. It is important to clarify the difference between remission and "curing" or "reversing" diabetes. When a patient has an early cancer, and the surgical team is able to resect it with no increased risk of a future recurrence, that is a cure. When a patient can maintain their glucose (HbA1c < 7.0% for many) without any medication, they are at goal. If this HbA1c (<6.5%) is maintained with normal glucose values for at least 3 months without any diabetes medication, this person has achieved "diabetes remission."[1] This is an important differentiation.

   Most often this is achieved via significant dietary modification accompanied by substantial weight loss. The ability to maintain the benefit from interventions that helped a person achieve their glucose goals lasts only as long as the intervention's effects persist. Thus, if the person gains weight, it is fair to assume their diabetes will return. They are at increased risk for recurrence for the rest of their life and will want to maintain the intervention to keep their diabetes in remission.

   In this case study, it is best to inform the patient that his condition can be controlled without medications, but a "cure" is not a realistic or attainable goal.

2. For a patient who is newly diagnosed and just starting the education process, a continuous glucose monitor (CGM) can be an invaluable tool. By providing a patient with clear glucose goals, and then having them see how their glucose responds to diet and daily activities, with immediate feedback from a CGM, we can help inform effective change. For example, a patient might learn how much their morning latte increases their blood sugar. Or they can recognize that if they walk their dog their glucose improves. These "self-discoveries" help patients make changes on their own and may inspire them to explore the impact of other lifestyle modifications. Moreover, these "self-discoveries" are rooted in science, specifically cognitive behavioral therapy. Encouraging your patient to try different behavioral experiments with lifestyle modifications and then observe changes in their blood sugars is an excellent strategy to educate and empower your patients.

Including a CGM in your initial education process and referring patients to formal Diabetes Self-Management Education and Support (DSMES) training helps provide them with tools for success. DSMES has been shown to have substantial benefits for people with diabetes including a reduction in HbA1c, reduction in all-cause mortality, improved self-efficacy, improved coping, decreased diabetes-related distress, and improved quality of life.[2]

Sadly, less than 10% of people with diabetes attend diabetes education within the first year of diagnosis, consequently setting them up for failure.[3] The rates are even lower for people with Medicare, which is unfortunate as diabetic education is a covered benefit.[4] A referral, with positive reinforcement from the primary care clinician, is one of the best predictors that a patient will attend this important training.

Lifestyle interventions are a cornerstone of diabetes management. There is strong evidence that aggressive weight loss via very low-calorie diets can put type 2 diabetes in remission. The DiRECT trial was a very low-calorie diet study coordinated through primary care offices. Results showed that 46% of participants achieved diabetes remission at 12 months and 36% maintained remission at 24 months.[5] The ReTUNE trial recently attempted a similar very low-calorie diet plan in people with type 2 diabetes but lower BMI.[6] They found that a mean weight loss of 9% enabled 70% of people to achieve diabetes remission.[7]

An important thing to keep in mind is that all intensive lifestyle interventions, including very low-calorie diets, must be accompanied with high levels of support if they are to be successful. This requires a team-based approach that includes the health care professional (HCP), a dietitian, diabetes educator, and the patient's family and friends. At first, they may require more support to initiate major changes and then the amount needed will vary based upon patient needs.

3. The 2022 American Diabetes Association (ADA) Standards of Care for people with diabetes has an algorithm to guide pharmacotherapy for people with type 2 diabetes.[8] First and foremost, any pharmacotherapy should be coupled with therapeutic lifestyle change in conjunction with diabetes self-management education and support.

Until recently the initial pharmacologic management of type 2 diabetes mellitus (T2DM) was fairly straightforward; most patients were started on metformin. Metformin is generally safe, effective, and affordable. This process is evolving to support the selection of initial diabetes agents based on the patient's coexisting medical conditions. As per the ADA's 2022 Standards of Care, if a person has existing atherosclerotic cardiovascular disease (ASCVD), heart failure, or chronic kidney disease (CKD), other medications are appropriate initial choices, either with metformin or in place of metformin.[8] For example, if a person has known ASCVD, use of a GLP-1RA (glucagon-like peptide 1 receptor agonist), or an SGLT-2 (sodium-glucose cotransporter 2) inhibitor with proven cardiovascular benefit is recommended. Similarly, if the patient has either HFrEF (heart failure with reduced ejection fraction) or HFpEF (heart failure with reduced ejection fraction), an SGLT-2 inhibitor is preferred. An SGLT-2i is also reasonable if the patient has CKD, or if the estimated glomerular filtration rate (eGFR) is <30 mL/min, a GLP-1RA with known renal benefit can be used as an alternative.

An important concept when choosing an appropriate regimen is to identify how far the HbA1c needs to drop for the patient's diabetes to be at target. This is dependent on one's initial A1c and their A1c goal. We will address individualizing a patient's A1c goal in later chapters.

A loose rule when selecting medications is to expect an approximate 1% decrease in HbA1c per medication used. Many patients at diagnosis have significantly elevated A1c levels. Therefore, it would make sense for a patient to require more than one agent to achieve their glycemic goal. Unfortunately, many physicians have been reluctant to begin an aggressive multidrug regimen at the time of diagnosis. More commonly, patients begin a step-therapy approach, where one drug is started, titrated to maximum dose, the A1c is rechecked, and if the A1c is not at goal, another medication is added. This is akin to Dr. DeFronzo's previously described "treat to fail" practices.

An example of a potent initial regimen is metformin plus the dipeptidyl peptidase 4 inhibitor (DPP4i) sitagliptin. Patients whose first treatment was metformin and sitagliptin in combination achieved a 2.4% drop in HbA1c and more people achieved an A1c of less than 7% vs metformin alone.[9] Another example is the concurrent use of metformin, the thiazolidinedione (TZD) pioglitazone, and the GLP-1RA exenatide as initial therapy. Using the three medications together was more effective in lowering HbA1c and helping with weight loss than sequentially added therapies.[10]

4. Many studies have shown the benefit of intensive insulin therapy as the initial treatment of type 2 diabetes. These studies used either an intravenous insulin regimen at the time of T2DM diagnosis or a basal/bolus insulin regimen. The rationale of these early insulin strategies is to "rest the pancreas" and reverse glucotoxicity and lipotoxicity. Later it was found that this treatment allows for redifferentiation of the pancreatic beta cells.[10-22]

The goal of intensive insulin therapy is to quickly obtain glycemic control, have a period of stability for at least 2, but preferably 4 weeks, and then taper the insulin dose. Assuming this patient was taking full insulin replacement with both a basal insulin and a mealtime insulin, the approach would be to adjust the mealtime insulin first, reducing it by 50% for 1 week. This is repeated each week until the person is on 5 units or less of prandial insulin. If they successfully stop prandial insulin, the next down titration is their basal insulin dose. The approach is the same. Ideally, within 4 weeks the patient will have achieved glycemic targets and will no longer be on insulin. In previous studies of people with newly diagnosed type 2 diabetes who completed an intensive insulin protocol, 54% were able to go into remission at 1 year.[22] In other studies patients had sustained remission for as long as 6 years.[21]

Finally, bariatric surgery is an option for patients with diabetes whose BMI is greater than 35 kg/m². Studies have shown that patients who undergo a roux-en-y gastric bypass or gastric sleeve procedure are 5.9 times more likely to achieve diabetes remission.[23,24,25]

Case Summary and Closing Points

Diabetes remission is a goal wished for by many but achieved by few. The best chance for a person to achieve sustained diabetes remission is to get diagnosed with type 2 diabetes promptly and gain control quickly. Current evidence suggests that there are multiple ways to achieve diabetes remission. This affords clinicians multiple options for patient care. Options include an intensive very low-calorie diet, metabolic surgery, and initial intensive insulin regimen.

References

1. Riddle MC, Cefalu WT, Evans PH, et al. Consensus report: definition and interpretation of remission in type 2 diabetes. *Diabetes Care.* 2021;44(10):2438-2444. doi:10.2337/dci21-0034
2. Strawbridge LM, Lloyd JT, Meadow A, Riley GF, Howell BL. Use of Medicare's diabetes self-management training benefit. *Health Educ Behav.* 2015;42(4):530-538.
3. Powers MA, Bardsley JK, Cypress M, et al. Diabetes self-management education and support in adults with type 2 diabetes: a consensus report of the American diabetes association, the association of diabetes care & education specialists, the academy of nutrition and dietetics, the American academy of family physicians, the American academy of PAs, the American association of nurse practitioners, and the American pharmacists association. *Diabetes Care.* 2020;43(7):1636-1649. doi:10.2337/dci20-0023
4. Li R, Shrestha SS, Lipman R, Burrows NR, Kolb LE, Rutledge S; Centers for Disease Control and Prevention CDC. Diabetes self-management education and training among privately insured persons with newly diagnosed diabetes-United States, 2011-2012. *MMWR Morb Mortal Wkly Rep.* 2014;63(46):1045-1049.
5. Lean MEJ, Leslie WS, Barnes AC, et al. Durability of a primary care-led weight-management intervention for remission of type 2 diabetes: 2-year results of the DiRECT open-label, cluster-randomised trial. *Lancet Diabetes Endocrinol.* 2019;7(5):344-355. doi:10.1016/S2213-8587(19)30068-3
6. Al-Mrabeh A, Barnes AC, Irvine KM, et al. Return to normal glucose control by weight loss in non-obese people with Type 2 diabetes: the ReTUNE study. *Diabetes.* 2021;70(suppl 1):1184-P.
7. Diabetes UK Professional Conference. *Abstract A49 (P37)*; 2022. Presented April 1, 2022.
8. ADA Standards of Care for the person with diabetes. *Chapter 9: Pharmacologic Approaches to Glycemic Control.* https://diabetesjournals.org/care/article/45/Supplement_1/S125/138908/9-Pharmacologic-Approaches-to-Glycemic-Treatment
9. Reasner C, Olansky L, Seck TL, et al. The effect of initial therapy with the fixed-dose combination of sitagliptin and metformin compared with metformin monotherapy in patients with type 2 diabetes mellitus. *Diabetes Obes Metab.* 2011;13(7):644-652. doi:10.1111/j.1463-1326.2011.01390.x
10. Abdul-Ghani MA, Puckett C, Triplitt C, et al. Initial combination therapy with metformin, pioglitazone and exenatide is more effective than sequential add-on therapy in subjects with new-onset diabetes. Results from the Efficacy and Durability of Initial Combination Therapy for Type 2 Diabetes (EDICT): a randomized trial. *Diabetes Obes Metab.* 2015;17(3):268-275. doi:10.1111/dom.12417
11. Kramer CK, Zinman B, Retnakaran R. Short-term intensive insulin therapy in type 2 diabetes mellitus: a systematic review and meta-analysis. *Lancet Diabetes Endocrinol.* 2013;1:28-34.
12. Kramer CK, Zinman B, Choi H, Retnakaran R. Predictors of sustained drug free diabetes remission over 48 weeks following short term intensive insulin therapy in early type 2 diabetes. *BMJ Open Diabetes Res Care.* 2016;4(1):e000270.
13. Lean ME, Leslie WS, Barnes AC, et al. Primary care-led weight management for remission of type 2 diabetes (DiRECT): an open-label, cluster-randomised trial. *Lancet.* 2018;391(10120):541-551. doi:10.1016/S0140-6736(17)33102-1
14. Al-Mrabeh A, Hollingsworth KG, Shaw JAM, et al. 2-year remission of type 2 diabetes and pancreas morphology: a post-hoc analysis of the DiRECT open-label, cluster-randomised trial. *Lancet Diabetes Endocrinol.* 2020;8(12):939-948. doi:10.1016/S2213-8587(20)30303-X
15. Retnakaran R, Choi H, Ye C, Kramer CK, Zinman B. Two-year trial of intermittent insulin therapy vs metformin for the preservation of β-cell function after initial short-term intensive insulin induction in early type 2 diabetes. *Diabetes Obes Metab.* 2018;20(6):1399-1407. doi:10.1111/dom.13236
16. Ryan EA, Imes S, Wallace C. Short-term intensive insulin therapy in newly diagnosed type 2 diabetes. *Diabetes Care.* 2004;27(5):1028-1032.
17. Chandra ST, Priya G, Khurana ML, et al. Comparison of gliclazide with insulin as initial treatment modality in newly diagnosed type 2 diabetes. *Diabetes Technol Ther.* 2008;10(5):363-368.

18. Weng J, Li Y, XU W, et al. Effect of intensive insulin therapy on beta-cell function and glycaemic control in patients with newly diagnosed type 2 diabetes: a multicentre randomised parallel-group trial. *Lancet.* 2008;371(9626):1753-1760.
19. Li Y, Xu W, Liao Z, et al. Induction of long-term glycemic control in newly diagnosed type 2 diabetic patients is associated with improvement of beta-cell function. *Diabetes Care.* 2004;27(11):2597-2602.
20. Hu Y, Li L, Xu Y, et al. Short-term intensive therapy in newly diagnosed type 2 diabetes partially restores both insulin sensitivity and beta cell function in subjects with long-term remission. *Diabetes Care.* 2011;34(8):1848-1853.
21. Shubrook JH, Jones SA. Basal-bolus analogue insulin therapy as initial treatment of type 2 diabetes mellitus: a case series. *Insulin.* 2010;5:100-105.
22. Presswala L, Shubrook JH. Intensive insulin therapy as the primary treatment of type 2 diabetes. *Clin Diabetes.* 2011;29(4):151-153.
23. Shubrook JH, Sathananthan A, Nakazawa M, Patel N, Mehta RJ, Schwartz FL. Inspire diabetes: a pulse of basal bolus analog insulin as the first treatment of T2DM. Presented at the American Diabetes Association Scientific Sessions 2014, San Francisco CA. LB-95 Poster.
24. Sheng B, Truong K, Spitler H, Zhang L, Tong X, Chen L. The long-term effects of bariatric surgery on type 2 diabetes remission, microvascular and macrovascular complications, and mortality: a systematic review and meta-analysis. *Obes Surg.* 2017;27(10):2724-2732. doi:10.1007/s11695-017-2866-4
25. Mingrone G, Panunzi S, De Gaetano A, et al. Metabolic surgery versus conventional medical therapy in patients with type 2 diabetes: 10-year follow-up of an open-label, single-centre, randomised controlled trial. *Lancet.* 2021;397(10271):293-304. doi:10.1016/S0140-6736(20)32649-0

Case 2. Develop Your Diabetes Care Team

"I am doing everything I can."

A 48-year-old Hispanic woman presents to establish as a new patient. She recently moved to the area to help her sister who is chronically ill. She has diabetes and wants to make sure she can get her lab work done. She was originally diagnosed with type 2 diabetes at age 38, but the year after she was diagnosed, she "got sick" and was told she had become type 1. She tries "really hard" to control her diabetes; "No one else is going to do it for me."

Her last doctor said she was his "model patient." She would get her labs done before each appointment, so she knew "what she was dealing with." She takes her shoes off at every appointment, and she sees the podiatrist quarterly. She makes sure to get her eyes examined annually. So far, she has not developed any complications.

She takes insulin NPH (neutral protamine Hagedorn) 12 units each morning, and 18 units before dinner. She knows how to count carbs and uses 1 unit of regular insulin for every 10 g of carbs with each meal. She also uses a correction dose of 1 unit for every 30 mg/dL that her glucose is above her goal of 120 mg/dL. She checks her glucose 4 to 7 times per day so she can "stay on top if it." She occasionally has lows if she eats less than she thought she would or if she miscounts her carbs, but she fixes that with some juice or glucose gel. She has not had any recent severe lows, but she has a glucagon pen just in case. She has never had DKA.

Med HX: type 1 diabetes 9 years, hypothyroidism 6 years.

Medications: NPH and R insulin as above, levothyroxine 75 µg daily, daily vitamin

Allergies: none

Family Medical History: sister with degenerative joint disease (DJD) hips and knees, no family history (FH) of diabetes.

Social History: no tobacco, no alcohol, and no recreational drug use. She lives with her sister, works as EMS (emergency medical service) operator.

Physical Exam: Ht. 5′5″, Wt. 134 lb, BMI 22.3, T 98.9, P 88, R 15

GEN: in no distress

HEENT: normal including thyroid exam

CV: normal

RESP: normal

Skin: vitiligo noted on neck and arms

Extremities: normal diabetes foot exam—pulse, skin, sensation to monofilament

Otherwise: normal exam

Labs: HbA1c 6.1%

Glucose Readings:

Fingerstick Glucose	Fasting	Prelunch	Predinner	Bedtime
	162	104	142	132
	64	189	108	111
	108	100	198	140
	88	167	130	143
	96	140	182	92
	58	190	90	137
	148	98	184	76

 CASE QUESTIONS

1. What should be the initial approach to the patient?
2. What resources are available to support her?
3. What resources are available to her health care team?

 ANSWERS AND EXPLANATIONS

1. This patient has latent autoimmune diabetes of the adult (LADA), a form of type 1 diabetes. It is very important that she knows what type of diabetes she has to allow her to have the tools to best manage her diabetes. As a reminder, it is not uncommon for people with LADA to be initially misdiagnosed; a middle-aged adult presenting with elevated glucose but not in DKA is typically assumed to have type 2 diabetes.

   This patient is working hard to manage her diabetes. She is checking her glucose frequently, counting her carbohydrates, and calculating her insulin doses based upon her food intake and glucose levels. It appears that she has a good skill set. Acknowledging the effort, she is giving, and providing her with positive reinforcement is very important.

This patient seems knowledgeable about diabetes self-management and based on her HbA1c, her diabetes is well managed. However, it can be beneficial at an initial visit to get a more detailed sense of what her typical day entails. This would include the exact timing of her insulin doses, and whether they are consistent from day to day. You would also want to know the timing of her insulin doses in relation to her meals, the content of her meals, and when and how often she requires correction doses. This will help determine the adequacy of her carbohydrate ratio and correction scale. It can also be useful to learn when she is more physically active and if recurring life events impact her regular routine. Once the schedule has been determined, you should teach her the basic pharmacodynamics of her insulin products. This allows her to use insulin to better match her daily schedule and reduce her risk of hypoglycemia. While this may seem like a lot of detail, this information establishes the building blocks for an effective insulin regimen.

Depending on one's practice it may make sense to have a dietician or diabetes educator meet with the patient to obtain this initial information. It is important for the patient to know that this meeting is not about changing their diet. It is intended to help make sure their insulin doses are appropriate. Ideally, we would want the patient to complete detailed logs for at least 3 days prior to their appointment. These logs should include all food eaten, drinks consumed, insulin dosing and timing, and any physical activity or other relevant action that affects the patient's glucose. Whoever they meet with will have the opportunity to learn the patient's routine; their preferred foods, the accuracy of their carb counting, how effectively they are using their correction scale, and the precision of these calculations.

It is important for the patient to know the onset of action and peak activity of their mealtime insulin. The onset of an insulin helps the patient to understand the timing of the insulin dose with respect to their meals. This patient is using regular insulin as her mealtime insulin. Regular insulin has a typical onset of action of 30 minutes, and a peak activity of 2 ½ to 5 hours after dosing. The peak of an insulin preparation is the time range in which the person has the most active insulin working and is at the greatest risk of hypoglycemia. For her to match her insulin's activity she should be taking her insulin 30 minutes before her meals. Because of its delayed onset and variable duration of activity, mismatched timing of regular insulin doses may lead to early hyperglycemia followed by late hypoglycemia as the insulin's effect lasts longer than the meal. This is a key educational topic for the patient. She will need to know how to recognize if she is becoming hypoglycemic and be prepared to treat it. It is important for her to understand factors raising her risk for hypoglycemia, such as increased physical activity after her meal, or eating a smaller meal than expected (Table 3.1).

The newer human insulin analog and biosimilar insulins have a more rapid onset of action, and shorter time to peak activity. For example, insulin lispro has an onset as quick as 15 minutes. This means it can be taken up to 15 minutes before the meal. These insulins allow more flexibility in timing and can be fine-tuned based upon the glucose reading before the meal. If her glucose is higher before

TABLE 3.1   Key Components of Insulin Action[1-16]

Insulin	Brand Name	Manufacturer	Source	Time of Action (h)		
				Onset	Peak Effect	Duration
Glulisine	Apidra	Sanofi	Human analog	0.2-0.5	1.6-2.8	3-4
Lispro	HumaLOG	Lilly	Human analog	0.25-0.5	0.5-2.5	≤5
Aspart	NovoLOG	Novo Nordisk	Human analog	0.2-0.3	1-3	3 – 5
Insulin aspart	FIASP	Novo Nordisk	Human analog	0.12	1-3	3-5
Insulin lispro AABB	Lyumjev	Lilly	Human analog	0.12	1-2	2-4
Biosimilar lispro	Admelog	Sanofi	Human biosimilar	0.25-0.5	0.5-2.5	≤5
Regular	HumuLIN R NovoLIN R	Lilly Novo Nordisk	Human	0.5	2.5-5	4-12

the meal, she can take her mealtime insulin earlier to allow it to start lowering the glucose before the meal raises it. Conversely, if she is running a bit lower, she may want to take her insulin closer to the start of the meal to let the meal "get a head start." In general, it is safer to use these insulins before a meal rather than after the meal.

The patient in this case study is also taking NPH insulin as her basal insulin. Basal insulin is intended to mimic the continuous background insulin the pancreas produces. Basal insulin helps to regulate hepatic gluconeogenesis and maintain glucose stability between meals and overnight. Forms of basal insulin include several analog insulins including detemir, glargine, and degludec. These insulins all have a longer duration of action and a minimal peak effect. While NPH is used as a basal insulin, its activity is different from the long-acting analog insulins. NPH has a much shorter duration of action and more significant peak activity (Table 3.2).

Finally, the duration of the insulin lets indicates when it is ok to take another dose of insulin. Understanding this helps prevent a patient from "stacking" their insulin and putting them at a very high risk of hypoglycemia.

One of the most important things we can do for this patient is to answer any questions she has about her regimen and offer her tools that will help her better understand how she responds to her treatments. She is a great candidate for a continuous glucose sensor; using one will allow her to see her response to different types of food and further refine her insulin dosing.

TABLE 3.2	Landscape of Basal Insulin Options					
Insulin	**Brand Name**	**Manufacturer**	**Species Source**	**Time of Action (h)**		
				Onset	**Peak Effect**	**Duration**
Detemir	Levemir	Novo Nordisk	Human analog	3-4	3-9	6-23
Glargine	Lantus	Sanofi-Aventis	Human analog	3-4	None	Mean 24
Biosimilar Glargine	Basaglar Semglee	Lilly Mylan	Human biosimilar	3-4	None	Mean 24
Degludec	Tresiba	Novo Nordisk	Human analog	1	None	42
NPH	HumuLIN N NovoLIN N	Lilly Novo Nordisk	Human	1-2	4-12	14-24

2. A motivated patient who is taking charge of their diabetes can benefit greatly from management resources, especially if they make the work of diabetes easier. Examples include online apps that help calculate carbohydrate content of foods, insulin dosing, or both. In addition, we should let the patient know what technology is available to help them including continuous glucose sensors and insulin pumps. While these devices are not for everyone, we should make the patient aware of their choices, so they can make informed decisions for themselves. One useful free option is the diabeteswise.org website. This website helps patients walk through the technology choices and allows them to hear from the experience from others.

3. Effective diabetes care requires a team. All teams should include the medical professional, at least one other key staff member in the office (medical assistant, nurse, or other) as well as access to a dietitian, diabetes educator, case manager, social worker, and mental health provider. These professionals are resources for both the patient and clinician to help improve the management of this complex, chronic disease. Unfortunately, many primary care clinicians do not have this type of support or the time or experience to fulfill all of these roles. Unfortunately, many primary care clinicians do not have the time, experience or the necessary support to fulfill all of these roles. Often the patient can involve people in their life as team members. This could include family, friends, coworkers, and religious leaders.

Access to mental health providers is limited in many regions across the United States and globally. To address this lack of access, the ADA created an online directory of licensed mental health providers with competence in treating people with diabetes. HCPs can look for mental health providers in their state for in-person and telemedicine services by visiting https://professional.diabetes.org/mhp_listing.

Case Summary and Closing Points

Type 1 diabetes and its adult variant LADA are complex autoimmune conditions characterized by insulin deficiency. Day-to-day glucose variability is a real frustration for many people with type 1 diabetes. As such this patient's engagement in self-care should be highly commended. One way clinicians can address patient concerns around the complexities surrounding diabetes treatment is to recommend supplemental resources like some of the many technological tools available. Further, a clinician can offer an objective voice to interpret and assess the plethora of tools and information available.

References

1. Apidra (insulin gluline). *Package insert.* Sanofi; 2019.
2. HumaLOG (insulin lispro). *Package insert.* Eli Lilly and Company; 2020.
3. Novolog (Insulin Aspart). *Package insert.* Novo Nordisk; 2021.
4. FIASP (Inulin Aspar). *Package insert.* Novo Nordisk; 2019.
5. Admelog (Biosimilar lispro). *Package insert.* Sanofi; 2019.
6. Lyumjev (Insluin Lispro-aabc). *Package insert.* Lilly USA, LLC; 2021.
7. HumuLIN R (Regular Insulin). *Package insert.* Lilly USA, LLC; 2019.
8. NovoLIN R (Regular Insulin). *Package insert.* Novo Nordisk; 2012.
9. HumuLIN N (NPH). *Package insert.* Lilly USA, LLC; 2019.
10. NovoLIN N (NPH). *Package insert.* Novo Nordisk; 2012.
11. Levemir (Insulin Detemir). *Package insert.* Novo Nordisk; 2020.
12. Lantus (insulin glargine). *Package insert.* Sanofi; 2019.
13. Basaglar (biosimilar insulin glargine). *Package Insert.* Lilly USA, LLC; 2021.
14. Tresiba (insulin degludec). *Package insert.* Novo Nordisk; 2019.
15. Tuojeo (insulin glargine). *Package insert.* Sanofi; 2015.
16. SEMGLEE* (insulin glargine-yfgn) injection. *Prescribing Information.* Mylan Pharmaceuticals Inc; 2021.
17. Diabeteswise.org website. Accessed December 12, 2022. https://diabeteswise.org/#/

Case 3. Older Adults With Health Problems and Diabetes

"Are you giving up on me?"

An 84-year-old woman presents for a diabetes recheck. It has been more than a year since her last visit. She was reluctant to leave her home during the COVID-19 pandemic. She was diagnosed with type 2 diabetes 20 years ago. She believes she had "good control" most of the time. She received diabetes education when she was first diagnosed and made major lifestyle changes to prevent diabetes from "beating her." She hopes her current medications are still working for her. She is on a fixed income and would struggle to pay more for any expensive medications.

She has not been checking her blood sugar as much as she used to. It has become harder for her to perform self-monitoring of blood glucose over the past few years. She occasionally has an aide check her glucose if she feels "funny." This has been occurring more frequently in the middle of the day, especially if she skips her lunch. A nurse comes every Monday to prepare her medicines for the week. The aide helps make sure she takes her medicines when she is supposed to, but she is not there for all her meals.

She has been feeling more worn out than she used to, and her memory is not as good as it used to be. She tries to "keep her old bones moving" as best as she can with her walker. She has become more worried about her health since she saw her kidney doctor last week. He told her that her kidneys are not working as well as they were 18 months ago. Also, her eye doctor just told her that her macular degeneration is getting worse.

Med HX: type 2 diabetes 20 years, hypertension (HTN) 22 years, dyslipidemia 20 years, knee and hip osteoarthritis (limiting ambulation) 10 years; CKD4—newly diagnosed this year, dementia 6 years, requiring ongoing home health care

Medications: metformin 1000 mg bid, repaglinide 0.5 mg tid before each meal, valsartan 160 mg daily, HCTZ 25 mg daily, pravastatin 40 mg daily, donepezil 5 mg daily, acetaminophen 650 mg tid, calcium carbonate 1500 mg daily, vitamin D 1000 units daily, ocu-vits daily

Allergies: none

Family Medical History: sister with DJD hips and knees, no FH of diabetes

Social History: lives alone, widowed × 6 years, has in-home health aide, and visiting home health nurse once a week. Receives meals-on-wheels; eats 2 to 3 meals per day, needs assist for transfers; no tobacco, no alcohol, and no recreational drug use

Physical Exam: Ht. 5'5", Wt. 183 lb, BMI 31, T 97.5, P 72, R 15, BP 168/68

GEN: in no distress, obese, subtle head nod

HEENT: normal including thyroid exam

CV: regular, soft early diastolic murmur left sternal border

RESP: normal

MS: chronic joint changes in both knees, kyphotic

Ext: 1+ pitting edema B/L lower extremities, slightly raised shiny red-brown patches pretibial region B/L

NEURO: oriented to person, place, uncertain about year. Monofilament shows loss to light touch to all toes to mid forefoot. Vibratory loss to tuning fork

Lab Values:

Comprehensive Metabolic Panel	Value	Reference Range
Sodium	132	136-145 mmol/L
Potassium, serum	3.6	3.5-5.3 mmol/L
Chloride, serum	99	98-110 mmol/L
Carbon dioxide (CO_2)	29	19-30 mmol/L
Urea, nitrogen, blood (BUN)	45	7-25 mg/dL
Creatinine, serum	2.4	0.5-1.10 mg/dL
eGFR	25	>60 mL/min/1.73 m^2
Glucose, serum	72	65-99 mg/dL
Calcium, serum	9.9	8.6-10.2 mg/dL
Protein, total	7.1	6.1-8.1 g/dL
Albumin	4.3	3.6-4.1 g/dL
Globulin	2.8	1.9-3.7 g/dL
AST (SGOT)	35	10-35 U/L
ALT (SGPT)	27	6-29 U/L
Bilirubin, total	0.7	0.2-1.2 mg/dL
Alkaline phosphatase	68	33-115 U/L

Lipid Panel	Value	Reference Range
Cholesterol, total	180	125-200 mg/dL
Triglycerides	154	<150 mg/dL
LDL (calculated)	70	<130 mg/dL
HDL cholesterol	60	>40 mg/dL men; >50 women
Non-HDL cholesterol	120	<130

Other Labs	Value	Reference Range
HbA1c	6.2%	<5.7% (normal)
Urine albumin/creatinine ratio (UACr)	24 mg/g	<30 mg/g
B12	80 pg/mL	160-950 pg/mL

CBC	Value	Reference Range
White blood cell count	5.0	3.8-10.8 thousand/µL
Red blood cell count	3.6	3.8-5.10 million/µL
Hemoglobin	11.3	12.6-17 g/dL
Hematocrit	34%	37%-51%
Platelet count	246	140-400 thousand/µL

CASE QUESTIONS

1. What is the A1c goal for this patient?
2. What are safety concerns for this patient?
3. What treatment modifications are recommended?

ANSWERS AND EXPLANATIONS

1. This is an older patient with multiple comorbidities. She likely has a limited life expectancy. When treating diabetes in a chronically ill elderly patient, the goal should be to improve A1c levels while minimizing hypoglycemia and, if possible, reduce morbidity and mortality. Her measured A1c is 6.2% but this may be inaccurate, as she is anemic because of CKD. Her average glucose may be even lower. She is at substantial risk due to hypoglycemia.

   The ADA recommends consideration of loosened glucose goals in older adults and in those with significant comorbidities that limit life expectancy or increase the risk of hypoglycemia or sequelae from hypoglycemia. This patient has many factors that could put her at harm should she become significantly hypoglycemic. Her frailty, arthritis, vision impairment, and aortic insufficiency all make her a significant fall risk. She has a cognitive disorder that could result in missed or repeated doses of her medication. Needless to say, she is at very high risk for an adverse outcome from aggressive diabetes treatment.

   For this patient, it is best to target an A1c close to 8.0%. Our focus is to prevent hypoglycemia, and reduce her medication burden, while not letting the glucose climb high enough to cause immediate risk (Table 3.3).

TABLE 3.3	Glycemic Treatment Goals in Older Adults		
Patient Characteristics	**A1c Goal**	**Treatment Options**	**Warnings**
Healthy older adult	<7.5%	Almost any	Normal warnings
Independent but 2+ comorbid illnesses	<8.0%	Treatments that help comorbidities (SGLT-2i, GLP-1RA)	Watch for hypoglycemia, hypotension, and renal function
Short-term assisted living	No specific A1c Glucose targets 100–200 mg/dL	Insulin regimen common if staffing allows	Avoid chasing glucose
Skilled nursing assisted living due to ADLs	Avoid reliance on A1c Avoid symptomatic hyperglycemia and hypoglycemia	Basal insulin and DPP-4i Fixed ratio combination	No clear benefit from glucose reduction/ avoid complications of hyperglycemia

Adapted from ADA SOC. Older adults: standards of care in people with diabetes (Chapter 13). *Diabetes Care.* 2022;45(suppl 1): S195-S207.

2. There are many safety concerns here. Specifically, as it relates to her diabetes and treatment, she is not likely to gain improvement in quality of life or length of life from intensive glucose management, but she is at high risk for hypoglycemia or inability to provide for herself if she does experience hypoglycemia.

   Current problems and concerns as they relate to her diabetes:
   1. Advanced age: higher risk of hypoglycemia and acute kidney injury
   2. CKD: higher risk of hypoglycemia and acute kidney injury; less likely to clear medications
   3. Dementia: concerns about safety dosing medication, checking glucose, and being able to respond to hyperglycemia and hypoglycemia
   4. DJD lower extremities: limited mobility leading to increased risk for falls during ambulation
   5. Valvular heart disease/widened pulse pressure: risk for falls
   6. Symmetric sensory polyneuropathy-suspect metformin induced/provoked: risk for diabetes-related foot wounds and falls

   Other important considerations to keep in mind include depression and acute delirium. Symptoms of depression (eg, "feeling worn down," "memory not as good as it used to be") may overlap with other health conditions, such as dementia and polypharmacy. For example, depression and dementia share several overlapping symptoms including fatigue, memory problems, and changes in appetite. However, differences in the time course and progression of symptoms can help distinguish between the two diagnoses. Symptoms of sad mood or affect and the acute onset of fatigue, memory problems, and changes in appetite are likely to represent depression, whereas a slow onset of fatigue, memory problems, and gradual changes in appetite are likely to represent dementia. Similarly, an immediate or recent impairment in memory, reduced overall awareness, and impairments in recognizing people, time, and place are indicative of acute delirium with physical illness and potential drug toxicity. Conversely, the onset of these symptoms in dementia occurs slowly over months to years, without the presence of physical illness or drug toxicity. Lastly, to complicate matters, symptoms of hypoglycemia (eg, irritability, fatigue, decrease in recent memory) can mimic symptoms of all three conditions (see box on Glucose Readings). Thus, distinguishing between symptoms of depression, dementia, acute delirium, and hypoglycemia can be challenging. Clinicians should rule out these possibilities through physical examination, medical interview (including family history), diagnostic evaluation by a neurologist, and laboratory investigations. Failure to distinguish among these conditions in older patients is serious because of the long-term, life-threatening risks for complications, functional disability, hospitalization, and mortality.

3. There are a number of changes in her medications that should be made.

   First, her eGFR is less than 30 mL/min; therefore, metformin should be stopped. In general, metformin should be used with caution if the eGFR is ≤45 mL/min and should be stopped if the eGFR is <30 mL/min.[1] The major toxicity from metformin use is lactic acidosis. The risk is much higher in people with advanced CKD.

   Next, her use of a secretagogue needs to be reassessed. While repaglinide may be helping to control her diabetes, this medication must be dosed with a meal. It is possible that her episodes of hypoglycemia are because she is taking this but not eating at the same time. A better alternative is to take this medication only at her largest meal or when her meal is supervised by her home health aide.

She has safer treatment options. Replacing metformin and repaglinide with a DPP4i is a reasonable choice. This provides some mild postmeal glucose coverage but a much lower risk of hypoglycemia. Linagliptin is the preferred DPP4i for patients with advanced renal disease as it is not renally excreted and therefore requires no dosing adjustment. Another option is to use a GLP-1RA either once daily or once weekly. This might be a safer approach; it could be administered by the home health care staff and would not require the patient to remember to take the medication. GLP-1a's have a very low risk of hypoglycemia. Most of the GLP-1RAs are not renally excreted, so they are safe to use in patients with chronic renal disease (with the exception of exenatide or lixisenatide).[2,3] Theoretically, choosing a GLP-1a might be preferred over a DPP4i due to potential cardiovascular and renal risk reduction. However, GLP-1a's are expensive, and this patient is on a fixed income and may not be able to afford the copay for these medications.

Medications to avoid in this patient include metformin, sulfonylureas, meglitinides, and anything that is dosed more than once a day. SGLT-2 inhibitors would likely be ineffective given her current renal function. They also would place her at unnecessary risk due to volume depletion.

Case Summary and Closing Points

HCPs should always strive to provide the right treatment at the right time to the right patient. This patient has done well, but the risk-benefit ratio of her treatment is leaning toward greater risk. This is a good example of a situation wherein the best course of action is to deintensify treatment. This decision is made on the patient's age, functional status, life expectancy, and patient wishes.

References

1. American Diabetes Association. Older adults: standards of care in people with diabetes (Chapter 13). *Diabetes Care.* 2022;45(suppl 1):S195-S207. https://diabetesjournals.org/care/article/45/Supplement_1/S195/138920/13-Older-Adults-Standards-of-Medical-Care-in?searchresult=1
2. Exenatide. *Package insert.* https://www.accessdata.fda.gov/drugsatfda_docs/label/2009/021773s9s11s18s22s25lbl.pdf
3. Lixisenatide. *Package insert.* https://www.accessdata.fda.gov/drugsatfda_docs/label/2016/208471orig-1s000lbl.pdf

Case 4.　It Is About the Process Not Result

"High fives and smiley faces go a long way."

A 34-year-old woman presents to establish care. She has a history of polycystic ovarian syndrome (PCOS) and type 2 diabetes. She was diagnosed with PCOS during a time when she was having trouble getting pregnant. She began treatment with metformin and was able to conceive. She was diagnosed with gestational diabetes during her first pregnancy. Her diabetes was treated with lifestyle changes, and she delivered a healthy 9 lb 8 oz baby. She thought she had "pretty good control" during her pregnancy. Shortly after delivery she stopped taking metformin.

Four years later she was having trouble getting pregnant again and found out she developed type 2 diabetes. This was a surprise as she thought her diabetes had gone away. She resumed metformin and was once again able to get pregnant. She stayed on metformin during the first trimester but then needed insulin during the rest of the pregnancy. She received more comprehensive diabetes education during this pregnancy. She worked hard to stay in "good control" as she wanted to protect her baby. She delivered a healthy 7 lb 6 oz boy at term.

After delivery, she went back on metformin. She was done having children, so she had a copper intrauterine device implanted. She saw her primary care clinician once about a year after her second childbirth, but the visit was "not good." She briefly asked about her efforts to manage her diabetes and told her she needed to work harder to lose weight. She did not even tell her what her A1c was.

For the past 3 years she has just been getting care from a local walk-in clinic. They just refill her metformin. She hoped it was working but she is not sure because she stopped doing glucose checks a long time ago. She is worried that her blood sugar is not well controlled, because she became very depressed after her last pregnancy and gained a lot of weight since her last child was born.

Her goals for the visit are to:

1. Find out if the metformin is "working"

2. Get a refill on medication and supplies so she can resume self-monitoring

3. Find out what she can do to take better care of herself, so she can take care of her kids

Med HX: type 2 diabetes 4 years, PCOS 7 years, dyslipidemia 4 years, postpartum depression

Medications: metformin 1000 mg bid

Allergies: none

Family Medical History: sister and mom with T2DM; sister with PCOS

Social History: lives with her spouse and two kids; works as an aide at kids' school

Physical Exam: Ht. 5'4", Wt. 198 lb, BMI 34, T 98.6, P 72, R 15, BP 122/68

GEN: in no distress; obese

HEENT: normal including thyroid exam

CV: normal

RESP: normal

MS: normal

Psych: depressed mood, congruent affect

Derm: hirsute

Otherwise: normal exam

Her office glucose is 148 mg/dL 2 hours post lunch, point-of-care HbA1c is 7.9%

CASE QUESTIONS

1. What should be the initial approach to this patient?
2. What treatments should be recommended?
3. How can her concerns be addressed?
4. What follow-up should be recommended?

ANSWERS AND EXPLANATIONS

1. This patient has had a gap in her health care. This is likely multifactorial. Certainly, as a working mother with young children, time for self-care comes at a premium. Her depression is likely a factor contributing to self-care neglect. However, a negative experience with an HCP is likely part of the delay. As many as three-fourths of women have reported that they have been disrespected by their HCP when it comes to weight-related chronic diseases.[1] Further, only about 10% have approached their doctor for assistance in weight loss.[2]

    The first thing to do for this patient is to congratulate her for taking the lead on regaining control of her health. Providing this patient with positive reinforcement will get things moving in a positive direction. She should be commended on her desire to overcome obstacles and set goals. We can share that with an HbA1c of less than 8% on metformin alone, and with improved self-care efforts she is very likely to obtain excellent control of her diabetes. By offering encouragement and sharing information, we have an opportunity to help her reengage in her care without overwhelming or discouraging her.

2. This is the ideal opportunity for us to offer her choices, elicit her preferences, and develop a shared decision plan. It is a great time to reintroduce diabetes education (and refer if necessary) and reinforce effective self-management behaviors. It is important for us to recall that she has not had any diabetes education since her pregnancy. She is now the mother of two young children, who have a genetic risk for developing diabetes themselves. Therefore, the education should focus on taking care of herself and helping to reduce the risk of diabetes in her children.

    It is important to assess her ability to modify both her and her family's daily habits. For many patients, implementing changes in diet and physical activity that affect the entire family can be challenging. However, if the work is reframed to help improve not only her health but also her family's, it may be more appealing.

    It is generally advisable not to add any medications at the first visit. A better approach is to get her set up for diabetes self-management education and have her testing her blood sugar again. Rather than overwhelming her with fingerstick glucose readings, consider asking her to do a mixture of timing of the tests; some first thing in the morning, some before meals, and some after meals (90-120 minutes) or at bedtime. For the sake of simplicity, ask that she check 1 to 2 times per day during this exploratory period to identify glucose trends at different times of day. Having her do this while also keeping a food diary will provide important information about when her glucose climbs and allow for a more targeted treatment strategy.

When determining an appropriate treatment regimen, it is necessary to identify each patient's A1c goal. This is best accomplished via shared decision making with physician guidance. In this young, otherwise healthy patient, an HbA1c < 7% is reasonable. Almost any treatment will work to lower her A1c 0.9%. By asking the patient what factors impact her choice of treatment (cost, weight gain/loss, avoidance of hypoglycemia, need for injections, wanting to avoid medications entirely, etc.), a more directed therapy can be determined.

3. Our patient wanted to know if her medications were "working." If we consider that she has had glucose deregulation for 7 years and has an A1c of 7.9%, during a time of inconsistent efforts at self-care, and has no known complications, we can reassure her that she is still getting benefit from metformin. As noted earlier, she should be commended on her initiative. We have discussed self-monitoring strategies and will need to make sure she has the tools she needs to be successful. Finally, she wants to keep herself and her children healthy. Keeping the focus on her family may be the motivation she needs, with the caveat that she has to manage her own health to provide for her family.

4. Since this person was out of treatment for a couple of years, she should have an early follow-up to take advantage of her current motivation and investment. At today's appointment, we can order fasting lab work to assess her kidney function, lipids, and urine microalbumin. We can also help her coordinate her DSMES training. There are continual advances in diabetes and helping the patient keep up-to-date with all of the latest tools will help her incorporate diabetes in her life.

At her follow-up appointment in 2 weeks, we can review her fingerstick glucose log; we should have enough information to make informed decisions for any further changes. We can coordinate referrals for her diabetic eye exam, perform her annual foot exam, and update any necessary immunizations.

When she returns, it is essential to take the time to hear her story. Learn what she has discovered for herself about her own health. Let her explain her glucose logs and what insights she has. In many cases, there will be an improvement in readings once the person starts self-monitoring, from the process itself. This is a great opportunity to provide even more positive reinforcement like a "high five" or a smiley face on the patient checkout sheet.

Patients spend a lot of time each day making small and large adjustments to manage their diabetes. It is important for us to provide support for the "process" (monitoring, assessing, and drawing conclusions) as well as the "product (HbA1c)." Recognizing the *work of diabetes* really helps patients know that their time and effort are valuable. This recognition also lets the patient know that they have an ally in their provider, someone who is also invested in the process. Supporting the *work of diabetes* really helps people with diabetes stay motivated and engaged.

Case Summary and Closing Points

Lapses and setbacks should be expected. Part of the role of being a clinician is to help patients veer toward the right health course for them when they move astray. This patient has been successful in the past but has had a setback. When setbacks happen, and they will, be prepared to offer encouragement and not punishments or threats.

Believe in the patient's own abilities to get back on track. Be part of the answer. Ask how you can best be a support. In this case a "carrot" will be much more effective than a "stick."

References

1. Lee JA, Pausé CJ. Stigma in practice: barriers to health for fat women. *Front Psychol.* 2016;7:2063. doi:10.3389/fpsyg.2016.02063
2. Stokes A, Collins JM, Grant BF, et al. Prevalence and determinants of engagement with obesity care in the United States. *Obesity (Silver Spring).* 2018;26(5):814-818. doi:10.1002/oby.22173

Case 5.   Reengaging Your Patient

"Welcome back from your diabetes vacation."

A 54-year-old man presented for his diabetes follow-up. He needs a refill of his medications. He was first diagnosed with type 2 diabetes 5 years ago. When he was initially diagnosed, he was really motivated to take charge of his health. He maintained his HbA1c goal with lifestyle and metformin alone for the first 2 years. However, last winter was longer and colder than normal. As a result, he struggled to keep up with his healthy lifestyle interventions. He exercised less and started snacking more at night.

He has a meter but has not done glucose checks in the past 60 days. He suspects he is running high because he is needing to urinate more frequently. He was worried about coming to today's visit out of fear he would get yelled at for losing control. His HbA1c 1 year ago was 7.1%. Today it has climbed to 8.6%.

Med HX: type 2 diabetes, HTN, dyslipidemia, gastroesophageal reflux disease, depression

Medications: metformin 1000 mg bid, sitagliptin 100 mg daily, glimepiride 4 mg daily, rosuvastatin 20 mg daily, lisinopril HCT 20/25 mg daily.

Allergies: none

Family Medical History: father—HTN, myotonic dystrophy type 2 (DM2), with retinopathy, CKD; mother with breast cancer. Brother with DM2, HTN, myocardial infarction

Social History: no tobacco, no alcohol, and no recreational drug use; lives with his spouse; works as an administrator at the local school

Physical Exam: Ht. 5′7″, Wt. 210 lb, BMI 32.9, T 98.2, P 92, R 12, BP 126/72

GEN: obese adult, in no distress

HEENT: normal including thyroid exam

CV: normal

RESP: normal

Otherwise: normal exam

Labs: fasting glucose 172 mg/dL, HbA1c 8.6% but all other labs are normal

CASE QUESTIONS

1. What is the best approach to this patient?
2. What can be done to reengage the patient?
3. What should be the follow-up plan?

 ANSWERS AND EXPLANATIONS

1. This is a common scenario. As previously discussed, diabetes is a self-managed lifelong, progressive condition that requires a significant amount of time and effort to achieve glycemic targets and maintain them over time. This patient knows that he is not doing well and, unfortunately, expects to be "yelled at" by his physician for his poor self-management.

   Rather than blame and shame it would be better to reframe our patient's recent experience as a setback rather than a failure. Remind him that with diabetes, as with all chronic conditions, perfection is unrealistic, and peaks and valleys are expected. The patient needs to know that his provider's role is to be an ally, and not to pass judgment. Not only does this instill confidence and trust in your relationship, but the patient is also reminded that he will have support when and if future setbacks occur.

2. Once a patient knows they are not going to be demoralized or punished for their lapses, they may open themselves up to engage in the process of problem-solving and shared decision making. When a collaborative tone has been established, it is helpful to ask the patient what worked for them in the past, and what may have changed or become a barrier to care. Together you can discuss effective interventions. This not only helps to set up a successful plan, but it also creates a framework for future interaction.

   This office visit may also be an opportunity to look at the "big picture" of this patient's overall health status. He has several chronic conditions and a very significant family history of complications related to those conditions. This can be an opportunity to discuss why it is important to manage his diabetes, dyslipidemia, and HTN from a risk-reduction standpoint. This can also be an opportunity to utilize shared decision making to inform treatment selection.

   If there are no contraindications, this is a great time to use a GLP-1RA either alone, or in combination with basal insulin. These medications have complementary effects; basal insulins lower the fasting glucose via its effect on the metabolism of carbohydrates, proteins, and fats, and the GLP-1RAs provide potent reduction of postmeal glucose excursions via increased glucose-dependent insulin secretion, decreased inappropriate glucagon release, and slowed gastric emptying. Further, by promoting brain-mediated satiety, the GLP-1RAs offset insulin-induced weight gain. These medications have shown strong potency and improved tolerability when used as a single fixed ratio medication.[1] At the current time there are two fixed ratio GLP1/basal insulin combinations available in the United States.[2,3] It is worth noting that these are branded medications; it would require that these be formulary-covered medication for people to be able to afford them. It should also be noted that these are only approved for use in patients with type 2 diabetes.

For many patients, this could also be an excellent time to use insulin for a limited duration to quickly achieve glycemic control. Once the patient is at their predetermined goal, insulin can be discontinued, and they can return to either their previous regimen or a new course of therapy. This strategy has several potential benefits. It promotes self-confidence as the person recognizes they can achieve their glycemic goals. It preempts the fear that once insulin therapy begins it will have to be maintained forever. It can also make insulin use more attractive should it be needed in the future. Some patients will want to maintain insulin use due to its simplicity and efficacy.

3. Regardless of which treatment is implemented, it is essential that our patient is provided frequent follow-up opportunities, or "touch points" to help him navigate back to his glycemic goals. Scheduling appointments every 1 to 2 weeks helps to ensure that each progressive step in treatment is achieved. After 3 to 4 visits, many patients will express that they feel like they have "got it" and are confident in their self-management skills. It is important for the provider to empower the patient at this time, reinforcing they can march forward capably on their own.

Since it will take 3 months to show a significant difference in HgA1c, initially it may be worthwhile to select a different outcome measure. Initially, the focus could be on fasting readings. Once these are at goal you may wish to focus on postprandial control. This would be a great time to consider the use of a CGM, as it can provide valuable positive reinforcement as the new regimen is started. The use of a CGM also offers the opportunity to remind patients about the impact their lifestyle has on their diabetes. It allows them to see improvements in their glucose control from physical activity and modification of dietary patterns. With this information they gain the ability to make informed decisions that help them feel more in control and empowered.

Case Summary and Closing Points

This is another patient who needs support and resources. He states he is going to be "yelled out." My guess is that he has already done that to himself. Let your patients know that setbacks are normal. The motivating factors or incentives for change for each patient will be unique, but in every case a clinician can promote change by inviting the patient to take an active role in determining the most effective treatment plan. Remind your patients that diabetes has many treatment options. If one does not work, try another. This message often helps long-term patients feel less stuck in their old treatment plans and the corresponding challenges they may have encountered.

References

1. Shubrook JH. Advances in T2D: focus on basal insulin/GLP-1RA combination therapy. Hot Topics in Medicine 8-2018. AND Blonde L, et al. *Curr Med Res Opin.* 2019;35(5):793-804.
2. Soliqua. *Package insert.* Approval 2016.
3. Xultophy. *Package insert.* Approval 2016.

Case 6. Handling Serious Comorbid Illness

"You need a diabetes pass."

A 64-year-old woman with previously well-controlled diabetes presents to discuss her new diagnosis. She recently learned she has stage 4 lung cancer. She just initiated chemotherapy and radiation treatment. She has not had much of an appetite and has been missing meals. She is worried about dropping too low if she takes her diabetes medications. At the same time, she is distressed if her blood sugar readings are high. She is uncertain what she should do.

Med HX: type 2 diabetes × 20 years, HTN 20 years, dyslipidemia × 25 years, stage 4 lung cancer

Medications: metformin 1000 mg bid, semaglutide 1 mg weekly, glimepiride 4 mg daily, atorvastatin 20 mg daily, lisinopril HCT 20/25 mg daily

Allergies: none

Family Medical History: noncontributory

Social History: 60 pk/y smoking history—quit last week, no alcohol, and no recreational drug use; retired and lives alone but has family nearby

Physical Exam: Ht. 5′7″, Wt. 165 lb, BMI 25.8, T 98.2, P 92, R 12, BP 116/62

GEN: overweight adult, tearful during exam; has lost 14 lb in the last 2 months

HEENT: normal

CV: normal

RESP: right side rhonchi noted with prolonged expiration throughout

Otherwise: normal exam

 CASE QUESTIONS

1. What should be the approach to this patient's glucose control?
2. What treatment modifications should be recommended?
3. What should be the long-term plan?

 ANSWERS AND EXPLANATIONS

1. Clearly this is a very difficult time for this patient. When patients get unsettling news or a life-threatening diagnosis, it is common for them to stop managing their chronic conditions. So, this office visit is a great opportunity to check in with the patient, help her come to terms with her current diagnosis, and help her see a path moving forward. If her prognosis is poor, this can be the time to discuss a lower intensity treatment for her diabetes. This is different from stopping all her medications and, in essence, signaling surrender. It is also different from maintaining intensive glucose control with the goal of reducing diabetes-related complications.

It is necessary to develop a plan that allows her to manage her diabetes without complicating her cancer self-care. For this patient, it makes sense to reevaluate her specific goals for treatment.

You may suggest not using her hemoglobin A1c to guide her diabetes regimen, as it may become less accurate during her illness. A fundamental aspect of care at this point is to minimize her risk for hypoglycemia as this poses a greater threat than the potential long-term complications of diabetes. Therefore, our initial focus should be on permissive moderate hyperglycemia. Since many chemotherapeutic agents can affect glucose, it is imperative that the provider touch base with the treating oncologist to determine which medication regimens and/or the use of corticosteroids are planned, so adjustments to our therapy can be made.

2. First, glimepiride should be stopped immediately. Use of a sulfonylurea with insufficient caloric intake places the patient at significant risk for hypoglycemia-related complications, including death.

   Second, stopping metformin is probably prudent. It is likely that because of chemotherapy-induced gastrointestinal side effects she will become volume-contracted, placing her at a higher risk of metformin-related lactic acidosis, which can also be life-threatening.

   Third, while semaglutide is a simple and effective treatment for her T2DM, appetite suppression is a common effect among GLP1-RAs. While this medication may help manage her blood sugar, it may also compromise her nutritional status.

   A reasonable glucose target for this patient is to maintain glucose values somewhere between 120 and 200 mg/dL. Keeping her blood sugar in this range will help prevent catabolic weight loss, dehydration from hyperglycemia-induced diuresis, and minimize her risk of infection.

   A reasonable treatment option for this patient is to stop all current diabetes medications and use a combination of daily basal insulin with correction insulin as needed based upon her glucose value and her appetite. Her basal insulin dose would be weight-based at 0.2 to 0.3 U/kg. Short acting insulin for correction is important for mealtime use and to address any episodes of severe hyperglycemia that may occur. This approach would allow her to manage her diabetes with minimal risk and minimal effort.

3. It may be too early to make a long-term plan. Our role now is to reassure the patient that we are still her ally and will support her throughout her cancer treatment. We can inform her that we will collaborate with her Oncology team and provide treatment recommendations that will manage her diabetes without complicating her cancer self-care. Once her response to treatment is known and her long-term prognosis is determined, a more specific plan can be developed.

Case Summary and Closing Points

While diabetes is a serious chronic and progressive disease, it may not always be the most urgent health condition at the time. When other serious illnesses come up, let the patient know that, in this case for example, the cancer is the priority, and you as the clinician will work diabetes treatments around the needs of the cancer treatment.

Note that this is very different than a course to not treat the diabetes at all. Again, the skill needed by the clinician is the right amount of treatment for a specific time and specific set of conditions. A loosened target and avoidance of medications that would exacerbate side effects of her other treatments may in fact be the best course of action.

Reference

1. ADA SOC. *Glycemic Management of Older Adults.* 2022. https://diabetesjournals.org/care/article/45/Supplement_1/S195/138920/13-Older-Adults-Standards-of-Medical-Care-in?searchresult=1

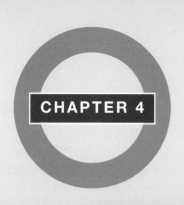

Navigating Diabetes Treatments

Introduction

There are many treatments for type 2 diabetes including 13 classes of medications. While this might be great in terms of having choices to individualize therapy, it is often overwhelming for the patient and the clinician. In truth, it is difficult to have a thorough understanding and working knowledge of all the medications available to treat diabetes. No matter what type of diabetes or the duration of the condition, therapeutic lifestyle change is central to management. For type 2 diabetes, most people will start with metformin and lifestyle change as initial therapy. The American Diabetes Association (ADA) now recommends specific type 2 diabetes treatments regardless of HbA1c in people with atherosclerotic cardiovascular disease (ASCVD), heart failure (HF), and chronic kidney disease (CKD). The following cases provide examples and situations for best placement of each treatment.

Case 1.   Therapeutic Lifestyle Change

"I do not want to take any medications."

A 36-year-old Asian woman presented for her annual physical exam. She felt well and had no complaints. She denied any new diagnoses, emergency room visits, hospitalizations, or medications. It had been a challenging year for her due to the COVID-19 pandemic, related to her work as a nurse in the pediatric ICU and having to coordinate home schooling for her two children.

About 4 years ago, her blood work showed that she had prediabetes, and this really scared her. At the time she made changes to her daily routines so she could get back to a normal glucose range. She began exercising more and reduced the amount of starches in her diet. She worked hard to stay healthy because both her mother and sister were taking medicines for diabetes. She wanted to do everything she could to prevent getting it herself. However, because of the COVID-19 pandemic, she had not been able to go to the gym and had not been as careful with her diet and had gained some weight.

She had her labs completed prior to this visit.

Med HX: dyslipidemia (6 years)

Medications: none and no OTC (over-the-counter) supplements or vitamins

Allergies: none

Family Medical History: mother and sister with type 2 diabetes; dad with dyslipidemia and coronary artery disease; no personal or family history (FH) of autoimmune conditions

Social History: no tobacco, no alcohol, and no recreational drug use; lives with her spouse; walks 30 minutes every day during her lunch break at work; eats a relatively traditional northern Chinese diet

Physical Exam: Ht. 5′6″, Wt. 152 lb, BMI 24.5, T 98.2, P 78, R 12, BP 112/70 (weight up 6 lb from last year)

GEN: in no distress

HEENT: normal including thyroid exam

CV: normal

RESP: normal

Otherwise: normal exam

Labs: nonfasting (90 minutes after eating)

Comprehensive Metabolic Panel	Value	Reference Range
Sodium	141	136-145 mmol/L
Potassium, serum	4.2	3.5-5.3 mmol/L
Chloride, serum	99	98-110 mmol/L
Carbon dioxide (CO_2)	26	19-30 mmol/L
Urea nitrogen, blood (BUN)	15	7-25 mg/dL
Creatinine, serum	0.64	0.5-1.10 mg/dL
eGFR	98	>60 mL/min/1.73 m²
Glucose, serum	185	65-99 mg/dL
Calcium, serum	9.9	8.6-10.2 mg/dL

Lipid Panel	Value	Reference Range
Cholesterol, total	158	125-200 mg/dL
Triglycerides	154	<150 mg/dL
LDL (calculated)	70	<130 mg/dL
HDL cholesterol	36	>40 mg/dL men; >50 women
Non-HDL cholesterol	122	<130

Other Labs	Value	Reference Range
HbA1c	6.8%	<5.7% (normal)
Urine albumin/creatinine ratio (UACr)	22 mg/G	<30 mg/G

CASE QUESTIONS

1. Does she have diabetes?
2. Is she overweight?
3. Why did her hemoglobin A1c not decrease despite 2 weeks of lifestyle modification?
4. What is the best test to diagnose her diabetes?
5. What are the best dietary interventions for her diabetes?
6. What resources are available to help her?

 ANSWERS AND EXPLANATIONS

1. Her HbA1c is currently in the diabetes range, but her nonfasting glucose is in the prediabetes range. While there is a strong clinical indication that she does have diabetes, it would be best to repeat an HbA1c to confirm the diagnosis. We advised her to repeat one of the following, an HbA1c, a glucose tolerance test (GTT), or a fasting glucose.[1] A repeat HbA1c 2 weeks later was 6.9%. This was very frustrating for her because she felt like she had taken control of her eating over the past 2 weeks.

   With two HbA1c readings above 6.5%, the diagnosis of diabetes can be confirmed. Given her family history of type 2 diabetes, and her lack of autoimmune disease, type 2 diabetes is most likely. Monogenic diabetes is also a possibility given a strong family history of diabetes, but you would not expect to see diabetic dyslipidemia (high trigs, low HDL [high-density lipoprotein]) in monogenic diabetes. With all of these factors considered she most likely has type 2 diabetes.

2. Evidence from the Centers for Disease Control and Prevention (CDC) and World Health Organization (WHO) illustrates that metabolic abnormalities can occur in lower weight individuals in some populations. Specifically, in Asian populations (Chinese, Japanese, Filipino, Indian, etc.), metabolic abnormalities can occur with a BMI of 23 kg/m². Consequently, the WHO has modified the BMI classification of weight in the Asian population.[2]

   BMI ≥ 23 kg/m² overweight
   BMI ≥ 27.5 kg/m² obese

3. This issue is important to clarify with the patient. The hemoglobin A1c is a good measure of glucose excursion over time. However, it is a measure of the glucose as it adheres to the hemoglobin molecule in red blood cells. While it may be reasoned from a patient standpoint that 2 weeks of lifestyle changes would lower the A1c, it is not realistic to expect changes that quickly. Her current readings of 6.8% and 6.9% are essentially the same given the specificity of the exam.

4. As mentioned in Chapter 1, there are four different ways to diagnose diabetes.[1,3] It can be diagnosed based upon elevated fasting glucose, elevated

hemoglobin A1c, with an abnormal GTT, or upon observation of significant hyperglycemia and typical catabolic symptoms (polyuria, polydipsia, polyphagia, and weight loss) of diabetes. With no single best way to diagnose diabetes, it is worthwhile to discuss the sensitivity and specificity of each diagnostic method[4] (Table 4.1).

TABLE 4.1 Glucose Ranges for Prediabetes and Diabetes Mellitus		
Normal	**Prediabetes**	**Diabetes**
Fasting glucose < 100 mg/dL	Impaired fasting glucose ≥ 100-125 mg/dL	Fasting glucose ≥126 mg/dL
2-h postmeal glucose < 140 mg/dL	Impaired glucose tolerance 2-h postmeal glucose ≥ 140-199 mg/dL	2-h postmeal glucose ≥ 200 mg Random PG ≥ 200 + symptoms
A1c < 5.7%	5.7%-6.4%	≥6.5%

Historically, the oral glucose tolerance test (OGTT) was the gold standard for diagnosing diabetes.[1,3] It has been the most sensitive assay for identifying glucose abnormalities (87.2% sensitivity, 77.7% specificity), but it does not have good reproducibility and has been shown to overestimate the incidence of diabetes. Further, it is difficult to get people to complete an OGTT due to the time it takes and the symptoms it may induce. Diagnosis via fasting glucose is less sensitive (70% sensitivity, 86.7% specificity), but the presence of fasting hyperglycemia correlates well with chronic hyperglycemia.[3]

Diagnosis via HbA1c is both sensitive and specific (sensitivity 87.1%, specificity 85.6%) and correlates well with diabetes-related complications.[3] It also does not require the patient to fast. However, HbA1c is reliant on the patient having a normal and stable hemoglobin. If a patient is anemic, has a hemoglobinopathy, or has recently lost, donated, or received blood, the HbA1c will be inaccurate for diagnosing or monitoring glucose control.[3] Finally, there is some evidence that there are ethnic differences in the HbA1c levels at the same glycemic levels.[5] Finally, some investigators have proposed combining the fasting glucose and HbA1c as a combined screen as this is as sensitive as the OGTT and more easily reproducible.[3]

While there are fewer supporting data, there is some evidence that the same tests and thresholds can be used to diagnose diabetes in children and adolescents[6] (Table 4.2).

Note. Positive predictive values are highly dependent on the prevalence of the disease in the population, whereas sensitivity and specificity do not vary by prevalence of the disease in the population. This explains the lower values for the positive predictive values.

TABLE 4.2 Sensitivity and Specificity for Current Tests for Hyperglycemia

Diagnostic Test	Sensitivity (%)	Specificity (%)	Positive Predictive Value (%)
HbA1c > 6.5%	87.1	85.6	8.7
Fasting glucose > 126 mg/dL	70	86.7	6.6
2-hour glucose (postmeal) > 200 mg/dL	87.2	77.7	4.8

5. As mentioned earlier, there is good evidence that diabetes can be prevented with lifestyle interventions.[7,8] However, the data are less conclusive on the use of life-style interventions for the treatment and remission of type 2 diabetes.[9-12]

The ADA provided updated guidelines for nutritional support in the management of diabetes in 2019.[13] This document described several core components of care. It identified medical nutrition therapy (MNT) as the evidence-based therapy provided by a dietitian. It also stated that all patients with diabetes should receive nutrition therapy, defined as treatment through the modification of nutrient or whole-food intake.

MNT has been shown to reduce HbA1c by up to 2.0% in patients with type 2 diabetes and 1.9% in those with type 1 diabetes.[14] In terms of nutrient recommendations, evidence suggests that there is not an ideal percentage of calories from carbohydrates, proteins, and fats for all people with or at risk for diabetes; therefore, macronutrient distribution should be based on individualized assessment of current eating patterns, preferences, and metabolic goals.[13] To be effective, MNT must be also highly individualized to the patient's cultural and family norms, work within the patient's means and preferences, and accommodate the individual patient's skill level in terms of diabetes self-management behaviors.[13]

A single nutrition therapy plan for all of diabetes may seem "too generic." There are a number of factors that should be considered when providing nutrition therapy to help to individualize advice to the patient and their needs:

1. What type of diabetes does the person have?
2. What role do food and nutrition play in the person's culture and religion?
3. What is the patient's living situation?
4. What financial and food resources are available for the patient?
5. Who does the person eat with, and who prepares the food?
6. Are there other medical problems that would complicate the recommendations (for example, heart failure, ASCVD, disorder eating) for this person?

A dietary plan that may at first seem simple may become daunting when these factors are taken into consideration. The true complexity of one's dietary practices is one of the many reasons that people with diabetes benefit from a diabetes self-management education and support (DSMES) program. This comprehensive training with the patient (and often family members as well) requires time, attention, and in-depth knowledge. Unfortunately, primary care clinicians typically lack the time and resources to adequately provide this level of support. A strong recommendation to seek the guidance of a dietitian or diabetes care and education care specialist can help the patient get the personalized help that they need to effectively manage their diabetes.

The goals of nutrition therapy are seen in Table 4.3.

TABLE 4.3   ADA 2019 Consensus Statement: Goals of Nutrition Therapy
1. To promote and support healthful eating patterns, emphasizing a variety of nutrient-dense foods in appropriate portion sizes, in order to improve overall health and specifically to:
a. Improve A1c, blood pressure, and cholesterol levels (goals differ for individuals based on age, duration of diabetes, health history, and other present health conditions)
2. Further recommendations for individualization of goals can be found in the ADA Standards of Medical Care in Diabetes
a. Achieve and maintain body weight goals
b. Delay or prevent complications of diabetes
c. To address individual nutrition needs based on personal and cultural preferences, health literacy and numeracy, access to healthful food choices, willingness, and ability to make behavioral changes, as well as barriers to change
d. To maintain the pleasure of eating by providing positive messages about food choices while limiting food choices only when indicated by scientific evidence
e. To provide the individual with diabetes with practical tools for day-to-day meal planning

Specific fundamental MNT teaching points include the following:

1. Assess the patient's cultural and family norms before advising on dietary plans. Working with a patient's heritage diet can help manage chronic metabolic conditions more effectively.
2. The ideal amount of carbohydrates is unknown. The 130 g/d of carbohydrates needed for brain function can be provided from the diet, but these can also be produced from the body's normal physiologic processes. Therefore, the previous thought that this was a minimum number of carbohydrates needed in a diet no longer applies. Lower carbohydrate diets are likely to be beneficial for most people with type 2 diabetes.
3. The quality of carbohydrates is important and can have a major impact on glycemic excursions. Whole-food sources should be encouraged as this will produce increased fiber content as well.
4. Fiber content is helpful not only for glucose control, but fiber intake has also been associated with reduced mortality. A minimum of 14 g of fiber should be consumed for every 1000 kcals ingested.
5. Fat should be 20% to 35% of all calories. Trans fats should be eliminated from the diet, and saturated fats should be limited.
6. Higher protein calories may improve weight loss but should be focused on plant sources whenever possible. Restricting protein in people with CKD is no longer recommended for most patients.
7. Patients with CKD will benefit from switching to a plant-based diet.

Case Summary and Closing Points

Type 2 diabetes is a chronic metabolic condition that is largely influenced by daily activities. While most people will need medication to treat their diabetes, there is strong evidence that lifestyle activities can play a large role in diabetes prevention and management. As such, it is important for clinicians to be knowledgeable about what programs have had the most success and how to help coach the patient to engage in these programs. Most clinicians engage a team to help with education including a certified diabetes education and care specialist and a dietitian. Equally important, any lifestyle change has to be a lifelong change, so it is also key to build in methods to sustain these changes.

References

1. American Diabetes Association. Standards of Medical Care 2022. Classification and Diagnosis and of Diabetes. 2022. https://diabetesjournals.org/care/article/45/Supplement_1/S17/138925/2-Classification-and-Diagnosis-of-Diabetes
2. WHO Expert Consultation. Appropriate body-mass index for Asian populations and its implications for policy and intervention strategies. *Lancet*. 2004;363(9403):157-163. Erratum in: *Lancet*. 2004;363(9412):902. doi:10.1016/S0140-6736(03)15268-3
3. Barr RG, Nathan DM, Meigs JB, Singer DE. Tests of glycemia for the diagnosis of type 2 diabetes mellitus. *Ann Intern Med*. 2002;137(4):263-272. doi:10.7326/0003-4819-137-4-200208200-00011
4. Colagiuri S, Lee CMY, Wong TY, Balkau B, Shaw JE, Borch-Johnsen K; DETECT-2 Collaboration Writing Group. Glycemic thresholds for diabetes-specific retinopathy: implications for diagnostic criteria for diabetes. *Diabetes Care*. 2011;34(1):145-150.
5. Wolffenbuttel BHR, Herman WH, Gross JL, Dharmalingam M, Jiang HH, Hardin DS. Ethnic differences in glycemic markers in patients with type 2 diabetes. *Diabetes Care*. 2013;36(10):2931-2936. doi:10.2337/dc12-2711
6. Vijayakumar P, Nelson RG, Hanson RL, Knowler WC, Sinha M. HbA1c and the prediction of type 2 diabetes in children and adults. *Diabetes Care*. 2017;40(1):16-21. doi:10.2337/dc16-1358
7. The Diabetes Prevention Program (DPP) Research Group. Reduction in the incidence of type 2 diabetes with lifestyle intervention or metformin. *N Engl J Med*. 2002;346(6):393-403.
8. Eriksson J, Lindstrom J, Valle T, et al. Prevention of Type II diabetes in subjects with impaired glucose tolerance: the Diabetes Prevention Study (DPS) in Finland. Study design and 1-year interim report on the feasibility of the lifestyle intervention programme. *Diabetologia*. 1999;42(7):793-801.
9. Pan XR, Li GW, Hu YH, et al. Effects of diet and exercise in preventing NIDDM in people with impaired glucose tolerance: the Da Qing IGT and diabetes study. *Diabetes Care*. 1997;20(4):537-544.
10. Look AHEAD Research Group; Pi-Sunyer X, Blackburn G, Brancati FL, et al. Reduction in weight and cardiovascular disease risk factors in individuals with type 2 diabetes: one-year results of the look AHEAD trial. *Diabetes Care*. 2007;30(6):1374-1383. doi:10.2337/dc07-0048
11. Lean MEJ, Leslie WS, Barnes AC, et al. Durability of a primary care-led weight-management intervention for remission of type 2 diabetes: 2-year results of the DiRECT open-label, cluster-randomised trial. *Lancet Diabetes Endocrinol*. 2019;7(5):344-355. ISSN 2213-8587 doi:10.1016/S2213-8587(19)30068-3.
12. Evert AB, Boucher JL, Cypress M, et al. Nutrition therapy recommendations for the management of adults with diabetes. *Diabetes Care*. 2013;36(11):3821-3842. doi:10.2337/dc13-2042_
13. Evert AB, Dennison M, Gardner CD, et al. Nutrition therapy for adults with diabetes or prediabetes: a consensus report. *Diabetes Care*. 2019;42(5):731-754. doi:10.2337/dci19-0014
14. Franz MJ, MacLeod J, Evert A, et al. Academy of Nutrition and Dietetics Nutrition practice guideline for type 1 and type 2 diabetes in adults: systematic review of evidence for medical nutrition therapy effectiveness and recommendations for integration into the nutrition care process. *J Acad Nutr Diet*. 2017;117(10):1659-1679.

Case 2. Best Practices With Metformin Therapy

"Is metformin going to hurt my kidneys?"

A 38-year-old man presents for a second opinion about his diagnosis of diabetes and recommendations for treatment if needed. He was diagnosed with prediabetes 4 years ago at an employee health fair. At the time he was given information about weight loss and the Diabetes Prevention Program. However, due to his busy schedule he was unable to make any major changes in his diet and in fact, had gained weight since then. This past year he learned that his glucose values climbed and were in the diabetes range. Subsequently, he was referred for diabetes education and given a prescription for metformin 1000 mg twice daily. He was reluctant to start the medication because he had friends who had "all kinds of problems" with this medication and his brother-in-law had to stop it because "metformin hurt his kidneys."

His goal for today's visit is he would like to confirm his diagnosis and wants to know if he really needs to take metformin. His HbA1c 1 year ago was 6.8%. He has not been monitoring his glucose. He has not been a diabetes educator yet.

Med HX: type 2 diabetes mellitus (1 year), hypertension (1 year), dyslipidemia (4 years)

Medications: metformin 1000 mg bid (not taking), enalapril 2.5 mg daily, pravastatin 40 mg daily (not taking)

Allergies: none

Family Medical History: obesity is present among all immediate family members; dad has high cholesterol and type 2 diabetes; mom is deceased from a stroke

Social History: no tobacco, no alcohol, and no recreational drug use; lives with his spouse and two kids, ages 3 and 5; works at the city facilities department; no regular physical activity outside of work and playing with his kids; does not follow any diet, but his wife says he is picky; eats sandwiches at most meals.

Physical Exam: Ht. 5'9", Wt. 200 lb, BMI 29.5, T 97.7, P 78, R 12, BP 132/78

GEN: overweight adult, in no distress

HEENT: normal including thyroid exam

CV: normal

RESP: normal

Diabetes foot exam: normal pulses, no calluses, or skin breakdown, normal sensation to monofilament

Otherwise: normal exam

Fasting Labs:

Comprehensive Metabolic Panel	Value	Reference Range
Sodium	141	136-145 mmol/L
Potassium, serum	4.2	3.5-5.3 mmol/L
Chloride, serum	99	98-110 mmol/L
Carbon dioxide (CO_2)	26	19-30 mmol/L
Urea nitrogen, blood (BUN)	15	7-25 mg/dL
Creatinine, serum	0.64	0.5-1.10 mg/dL
eGFR	98	>60 mL/min/1.73 m^2
Glucose, serum	185	65-99 mg/dL
Calcium, serum	9.9	8.6-10.2 mg/dL
Protein, total	7.1	6.1-8.1 g/dL
Albumin	4.3	3.6-4.1 g/dL
Globulin	2.8	1.9-3.7 g/dL
AST (SGOT)	50	10-35 U/L
ALT (SGPT)	56	6-29 U/L
Bilirubin, total	0.7	0.2-1.2 mg/dL
Alkaline phosphatase	100	33-115 U/L

Lipid Panel	Value	Reference Range
Cholesterol, total	268	125-200 mg/dL
Triglycerides	244	<150 mg/dL
LDL (calculated)	180	<130 mg/dL
HDL cholesterol	32	>40 mg/dL men; >50 women
Non-HDL cholesterol	236	<130

Other Labs	Value	Reference Range
HbA1c	8.8%	<5.7% (normal)
Urine albumin/creatinine ratio (UACr)	108 mg/G	<30 mg/g

CBC	Value	Reference Range
White blood cell count	8.8	3.8-10.8 thousand/µL
Red blood cell count	4.8	3.8-5.10 million/µL
Hemoglobin	14.3	12.6-17 g/dL
Hematocrit	48	37%-51%
MCV (mean corpuscular volume)	91	80-100 fL
MCH (mean corpuscular hemoglobin)	29.9	27-33 pg
MCHC (mean corpuscular hemoglobin concentration)	32.9	32-36 g/dL
RDW (red cell distribution width)	12.7	1%-15%
Platelet count	336	140-400 thousand/µL

CASE QUESTIONS

1. Does he have diabetes? How can this diagnosis be confirmed?
2. Does he need to take metformin? If yes, how should it be prescribed to a first-time user?
3. What are the warnings with metformin? Does metformin injure the kidneys?
4. What other treatments can be recommended to this patient?

 ANSWERS AND EXPLANATIONS

1. Typically, the diagnosis of diabetes requires two tests separated by time in an asymptomatic person. This patient had an HbA1c 1 year ago of 6.8%. His current HbA1c is 8.8% and his current fasting glucose is 185 mg/dL. No further testing is needed to confirm that this patient has diabetes. He has had at least three tests demonstrating an abnormal glucose and the last three tests were within diabetes range values. He has type 2 diabetes that has progressed further during this past year.

2. This patient has type 2 diabetes and at least one complication related to his diabetes. We need to initiate a treatment regimen immediately to control his blood sugars and limit future sequelae. His hypertension and hyperlipidemia place him at high risk for renal and cardiovascular disease (CVD); the presence of microalbuminuria is a predictor of worse outcomes for both disease states.[1]

   Metformin is the most common treatment initiated for type 2 diabetes as it is typically safe, inexpensive, and weight neutral. Starting metformin, in addition to therapeutic lifestyle change, is a common and reasonable first step for treatment with patients such as this. It is likely, based on his current HbA1c and the presence of microalbuminuria, he will require additional medications; however, metformin should be part of the regimen, nonetheless.

   Patients starting metformin often experience mild gastrointestinal (GI) side effects including nausea and diarrhea. These can be minimized by starting with a dose of 500 mg in the evening. Once the patient is tolerating this without side effects, the dose can be increased to 500 mg bid (breakfast and dinner). Subsequently this can be increased to 500 mg in the AM, and 1000 mg in the PM, and then 1000 mg bid. It is important to maintain each dose until the patient tolerates it without side effects. Since metformin will be a long-term medication, it makes sense to take time to work up to the target dose[2] to assure tolerability and to improve compliance. Since type 2 diabetes is progressive, every attempt should be made to find a dose that this patient can tolerate so metformin can be part of his treatment plan.

   An alternative approach is to use extended-release metformin. This has less side effects and can be dosed once daily. The same approach to titration is utilized when using the extended-release formulation. It is worth noting that approximately 18% of people will not tolerate a therapeutic dose of metformin and will require other treatment regimens.

3. Metformin has several warnings and precautions. Some people can develop B_{12} deficiency and a related peripheral neuropathy from metformin.[3] Doses of metformin >1500 mg daily can reduce vitamin B_{12} levels 14% to 30%. For most people this does not lead to clinical B_{12} deficiency.[4] However, it is recognized that the development of B_{12} deficiency is directly associated with the duration of treatment with metformin.[5] While there is no consensus in terms of screening, any person on long-term metformin should have vitamin B_{12} levels tested on a regular basis and take supplemental B_{12} if they are deficient or if they have symptomatic peripheral sensory neuropathy.

   The most serious warning with metformin is the risk of lactic acidosis.[6] This is primarily based on the occurrence of lactic acidosis with a different biguanide, phenformin that was removed from the US market in 1976.[7] Data suggesting an increased risk of lactic acidosis in metformin-treated patients with CKD are limited, and no randomized controlled trials have been conducted to test the safety of metformin in patients with significantly impaired kidney function.[8]

   However, the risk for lactic acidosis can be prevented in most people if metformin is avoided in patients with acute renal insufficiency, stage 4 and 5 CKD or conditions that predispose to reduced renal function, including cirrhosis, and heart failure. It is important to remember that metformin dose should be reduced if estimated glomerular filtration rate (eGFR) is less than 45 mL/min and it should be stopped if the eGFR is <30 mL/min.[7] Metformin is usually also stopped before elective procedures and during hospitalizations. This is due to concern about a reduction in kidney function (from the hospital illness or procedure) that can result in metformin levels building up if they cannot be cleared by the kidney.

   Patients often misinterpret the warnings regarding the use of metformin in the presence of severe renal disease, believing that metformin was the cause of renal dysfunction. It is important that patients know that metformin is not causing the problem, and there is no evidence that metformin is hazardous to the kidneys.

4. There are lots of options for this patient. First, it is very important to let him know that being an active partner in his diabetes management is important. This means we will be working together to address the lifestyle factors affecting his chronic health conditions including diabetes, hypertension, dyslipidemia, and albuminuria.

   Based upon his current metabolic panel and urinalysis, he has stage G1A2 CKD. This indicates normal renal function, based on his eGFR of 98 mL/min with the presence of proteinuria. Despite his normal eGFR, it is important to recognize that he is at higher risk of developing progressive CKD and cardiovascular events.[10]

   The 2022 ADA treatment algorithm lists specific recommended treatments based upon compelling comorbidities and indications.[9] The presence of albuminuria makes the use of an SGLT-2 (sodium-glucose cotransporter-2) inhibitor a good choice, independent of his HbA1c, since this class of medication has evidence for renal protective benefits. SGLT-2 inhibitors have been shown to reduce the progression of diabetic kidney disease (both decline in eGFR and increase in albuminuria), as well as lower the risk for end-stage kidney disease, death, and cardiovascular death.[11-13]

This patient could also take a GLP-1RA (glucagon-like peptide-1 receptor agonist). This will treat his hyperglycemia and reduce his cardiovascular risk. This class has many formulations including a once-daily oral agent, once- or twice-daily subcutaneous injectable agents, and once-weekly subcutaneous injectable agents.

These variations allow patients to choose medication based upon coverage and dosing preferences. Weight loss is a prominent benefit of this class of agents. A primary care–focused review outlines the additional benefits of these medications.[14]

Finally, there is a relatively new medication that is helpful to reduce albuminuria in diabetes-related kidney disease. Finerenone, a mineralocorticoid receptor agonist, has been shown to reduce albuminuria in these patients on top of standard of care described above.[15] Further, adding finerenone to standard of care will reduce progression to CKD and cardiovascular events.[16,17] This treatment has been added to the ADA and the Kidney Foundation treatment recommendations[9,18] (updated guidelines in diabetes will be coming out in late 2022).

Case Summary and Closing Points

While treatment options do change frequently, metformin is still the most common initial pharmacologic treatment for type 2 diabetes. Metformin can be a hard medicine to tolerate, so be prepared with suggestions to make it easier. It is also key to know when metformin should not be used as well as the common adverse effects, so they can be addressed effectively.

References

1. Chronic Kidney Disease Prognosis Consortium; Matsushita K, van der Velde M, Astor BC, et al. Association of estimated glomerular filtration rate and albuminuria with all-cause and cardiovascular mortality in general population cohorts: a collaborative meta-analysis. *Lancet.* 2010;375(9731):2073-2081. doi:10.1016/S0140-6736(10)60674-5

2. Young CF, Dugan J, Pfotenhauer K, Shubrook JH. Pharmacologic management of type 2 diabetes. Part 2. *Prim Care Rep.* 2016;22(11):129-139.

3. Kim J, Ahn CW, Fang S, Lee HS, Park JS. Association between metformin dose and vitamin B12 deficiency in patients with type 2 diabetes. *Medicine (Baltim).* 2019;98(46):e17918. doi:10.1097/MD.0000000000017918

4. Ting RZW, Szeto CC, Chan MHM, Ma KK, Chow KM. Risk factors of vitamin B12 deficiency in patients receiving metformin. *Arch Intern Med.* 2006;166(18):1975-1979. doi:10.1001/archinte.166.18.1975

5. Aroda VR, Edelstein SL, Goldberg RB, et al; Diabetes Prevention Program Research Group. Long-term metformin use and vitamin B12 deficiency in the diabetes prevention program outcomes study. *J Clin Endocrinol Metab.* 2016;101(4):1754-1761. doi:10.1210/jc.2015-3754

6. Package insert Metformin. Accessed 2022. https://www.accessdata.fda.gov/drugsatfda_docs/label/2017/020357s037s039,021202s021s023lbl.pdf

7. Gan SC, Barr J, Arieff AI, Pearl RG. Biguanide-associated lactic acidosis: case report and review of the literature. *Arch Intern Med.* 1992;152(11):2333-2336.

8. Inzucchi SE, Lipska KJ, Mayo H, Bailey CJ, McGuire DK. Metformin in patients with type 2 diabetes and kidney disease: a systematic review. *JAMA.* 2014;312(24):2668-2675.

9. ADA Standards of Care for the person with diabetes. Chapter 9: Pharmacologic Approaches to Glycemic Control. 2022. https://diabetesjournals.org/care/article/45/Supplement_1/S125/138908/9-Pharmacologic-Approaches-to-Glycemic-Treatment

10. ADA Standards of Care for the person with diabetes. Chapter 11. Chronic kidney disease and risk management: standards of medical care in diabetes—2022. *Diabetes Care*. 2022;45(suppl 1):S175-S184. https://diabetesjournals.org/care/article/45/Supplement_1/S175/138914/11-Chronic-Kidney-Disease-and-Risk-Management

11. Heerspink HJL, Stefansson BV, Correa-Rotter R, et al. Dapagliflozin in patients with chronic kidney disease. *N Engl J Med*. 2020;383(15):1436-1446.

12. Boehringer Ingelheim. *Jardiance® (Empagliflozin) Phase III EMPA-KIDNEY Trial Will Stop Early Due to clear Positive Efficacy in People with Chronic Kidney Disease*; 2022. Accessed April 2022. https://www.boehringer-ingelheim.com/human-health/metabolic-diseases/early-stop-chronic-kidney-disease-trial-efficacy

13. McGuire DK, Shih WJ, Cosentino F, et al. Association of SGLT2 inhibitors with cardiovascular and kidney outcomes in patients with type 2 diabetes: a meta-analysis. *JAMA Cardiol*. 2021;6(2):148-158.

14. Gotfried R. How to use type 2 diabetes meds to lower CV disease risk. *J Fam Pract*. 2019;68(9):494;498;500;504.

15. Bakris GL, Agarwal R, Anker SD, et al; FIDELIO-DKD Investigators. Effect of finerenone on chronic kidney disease outcomes in type 2 diabetes. *N Engl J Med*. 2020;383(23):2219-2229. doi:10.1056/NEJMoa2025845

16. Pitt B, Filippatos G, Agarwal R, et al; FIGARO-DKD Investigators. Cardiovascular events with finerenone in kidney disease and type 2 diabetes. *N Engl J Med*. 2021;385(24):2252-2263. doi:10.1056/NEJMoa2110956

17. Agarwal R, Filippatos G, Pitt B, et al. Cardiovascular and kidney outcomes with finerenone in patients with type 2 diabetes and chronic kidney disease: the FIDELITY pooled analysis. *Eur Heart J*. 2022;43(6):474-484. doi:10.1093/eurheartj/ehab777

18. TKF Guidelines. Kidney International Practice Guidelines. KDIGO 2020 Clinical Practice Guidelines for Diabetes Management in Chronic Kidney Disease. Accessed December 28, 2022. https://www.kidney-international.org/article/S0085-2538(20)30718-3/fulltext

Case 3. How to Select a Diabetes Medication

"Is this medication right for me?"

A 49-year-old woman presents to discuss treatment options for her diabetes. She was diagnosed 6 months ago. She found out that she had diabetes at the time of her annual gynecologic exam. She has always been prone to urinary tract infections (UTIs), and this year she was having frequent yeast infections. At diagnosis she completed diabetes education, and she was started on metformin. She has no problems taking metformin, but she is not sure what it actually does to help her diabetes. She has seen commercials about these new diabetes medications and is wondering if she is on the right treatment.

Med HX: type 2 diabetes mellitus (6 months), dyslipidemia (2 years), recurrent UTIs (10 years), recurrent yeast infections (1 year)

Medications: metformin 1000 mg bid, simvastatin 40 mg daily (not taking)

Allergies: none

Family Medical History: dad has high cholesterol and type 2 diabetes; mom has chronic pancreatitis and had uterine cancer

Social History: no tobacco, 1 glass of wine 2× a week, and no recreational drug use. She lives with her spouse and has two adult children ages 25 and 21. She works at a local law firm as a paralegal. She recently joined a gym and has been going 2 to 3 times a week. Prior to her diagnosis her diet was primarily fast food and frozen meals. She is working on reducing the starches in her diet and has changed to diet sodas.

Physical Exam: Ht. 5′7″, Wt. 200 lb, BMI 31.3, T 97.7, P 78, R 12, BP 132/78

GEN: overweight adult, in no distress

HEENT: normal including thyroid exam

CV: normal

RESP: normal

Diabetes foot exam: normal pulses, no calluses, or skin breakdown, normal sensation to monofilament

Otherwise: normal exam

Labs: HbA1c 7.9%

Glucose logs are as follows.

Chart of glucose logs:

	Monday	Tuesday	Wednesday	Thursday	Friday	Saturday	Sunday
Prebreakfast	136	145	158	124	156	112	143
Prelunch							
Predinner		112	168		123		
Bedtime							
Notes			Not sure why I am higher		Did the same thing as Wed but different response		

 CASE QUESTIONS

1. How would you advise this patient?
2. How do we distinguish between diabetes treatments?
3. What are some of the best combinations of medications?

 ANSWERS AND EXPLANATIONS

1. Helping patients control their diabetes can be very challenging. Part of that task involves the selection of medications. Clinicians can serve as advisors using their expertise to help patients make educated decisions. The challenge to clinician is helping patients to select medications that align with both the clinician's treatment strategies and the patient's priorities.

   Encouraging the patient to be actively involved in treatment is an important part of their success. In this case study, the patient can and should be congratulated for being inquisitive about medication options. Her desire to understand what metformin does to control her blood sugar provides her clinician with a valuable teaching opportunity. The scenario also affords her the chance to ask follow-up questions; ideally helping her to be more effective in her self-care behaviors.

Her clinician can provide her with valuable information about what she can expect from different medications, including HbA1c reduction, dosing, side effects, and beneficial effects. This will help her to make an informed decision about her treatment plan. While this may sound overwhelming to have to know all of these details at first, this approach will ultimately help to strengthen the bond between patient and clinician. Both feel great efficacy in the treatments when they see the expected response and feel like treatment is successful.

Items to discuss when reviewing medications with a patient:

Drug Action	Drug Dosing	Drug Side Effects
How it works?	How is it dosed?	What are the most common side effects?
What is the expected change in glucose? (fasting, postmeal)	How often is it dosed?	How can side effects be mitigated?
What are the extraglycemic effects?	What are the warnings?	
	What are the contraindications?	

2. The initial step in determining the most appropriate treatment for any given patient is to review the patient's glucose readings and discuss how they compare to your, the clinician's, treatment goals. Then, divide the medication options by cost, effects on weight, whether they can cause hypoglycemia, and finally what glucose parameter (A1c reduction, fasting glucose, postprandial glucose) they can expect to see change with each medication.

A review of all the currently available noninsulin medications, their glucose-lowering effects, side effects, and nonglycemic effects have been published.[1-3] They are summarized below.

Metformin: This medication works to downregulate gluconeogenesis in the liver. Its effects are on lowering the fasting glucose. It is inexpensive, not likely to cause hypoglycemia, and for most people is weight neutral.

Metformin has common side effects (GI—upset stomach, nausea, belching, and diarrhea) that for most people resolve over time. It is available both as a tablet or liquid. It comes in both an immediate-release formulation, which must be dosed 2 to 3 times daily, and an extended-release tablet, which is dosed once daily. The extended-release form is often preferred due to ease of dosing and has fewer GI side effects.

There is a reported association with metformin use ($\geq$1500 mg/d) and B_{12} deficiency.[4] Metformin should be stopped in patients who become acutely ill or hospitalized due to the risk for potentially life-threatening lactic acidosis. Metformin dosing is dependent on renal function; the dose should be reduced (or not started) if the eGFR is less than 45 mL/min and should be stopped when the eGFR is less than 30 mL/min.[5] Metformin is contraindicated in people who have or are at risk for lactic acidosis, advanced cirrhosis, or symptomatic heart failure.

Sulfonylureas: These medications stimulate the pancreas to secrete more insulin. This process is glucose independent—meaning the strength of a sulfonylurea is not influenced by the current glucose. They are most effective early in the disease course, affecting both fasting and mealtime glucose readings but become less effective over time. They are typically dosed 1 to 2 times daily. Because their effect is independent of glucose elevations, they can cause hypoglycemia. Their primary advantage is that they are inexpensive. Sulfonylureas are not weight neutral; many people experience a modest weight gain on these medications. They are not recommended in people at high risk for hypoglycemia, with advanced renal disease (glipizide is the preferred sulfonylurea if CKD is present), or if a patient has hypoglycemia unawareness. There is no evidence that sulfonylureas reduce major diabetes-related adverse events.

Meglitinides: Meglitinides are similar to sulfonylureas in that they enhance pancreatic insulin secretion, but their duration of action is much shorter. Like sulfonylureas, their effect is dependent on the pancreas being able to secrete insulin; hence, they are used early in diabetes treatment. They are typically used in conjunction with a meal; hence, their effect is on mealtime glucose only. Their advantage in comparison to sulfonylureas is that they are less likely to contribute to hypoglycemia if taken with meals. Some people choose to use them only for high-carbohydrate meals. They are moderately inexpensive and have a side-effect profile similar to sulfonylureas. They are not recommended in people at high risk for hypoglycemia, advanced renal disease, or if a patient has hypoglycemia unawareness. There is no evidence that meglitinides reduce major diabetes-related adverse events.

Dipeptidyl peptidase (DPP)-4 inhibitors: DPP-4 inhibitors are a good comparator to the sulfonylurea/meglitinides. DPP-4 inhibitors work by blocking the action of an enzyme that destroys the hormone incretin. Incretins inhibit glucagon release, decrease hepatic glucose production, and enhance insulin secretion in a glucose-dependent manner. This important detail means that they are not associated with hypoglycemia or weight gain. They are tablets taken once daily. While they are expensive, their advantage is that they are among the best-tolerated medications for diabetes. They are not quite as effective as other medications regarding glycemic control. There are rare side effects associated with the use, including severe joint pain, bullous pemphigoid, and an association with pancreatitis. Two of the DPP-4 inhibitors (saxagliptin and alogliptin) carry black box warnings regarding an increased incidence of hospitalization for heart failure. Linagliptin is unique among the DPP-4 inhibitors in that it can be used in patients with impaired renal function. This class has not been shown to reduce any cardiovascular or renal complications.

GLP-1RA: This is another class of medications that impact incretin levels like the DPP-4 inhibitors. However, this class has a few key differences. GLP-1RAs have a pharmacologic level change in GLP-1 levels and therefore they are more potent than the DPP-4 inhibitors and they also have more side effects. Specifically, they have a greater effect on satiety than the DPP-4 inhibitors. As a result, the GLP-1As help to promote weight loss. All but one of the GLP-1RA are given by subcutaneous injection. They are more effective than DPP-4 inhibitors, so there will be greater reductions in the fasting and postmeal glucose because they increase glucose-dependent insulin secretion but also reduce glucagon. Their most common side effects are nausea, bloating, and diarrhea. This can be minimized with slow dose titration. These medications are branded and expensive. They have warnings about pancreatitis and medullary thyroid cancer (this is an autosomal dominant genetic cancer that is extremely rare). GLP-1RAs should not be used in people with a personal or family history of medullary thyroid cancer or MEN-2 (multiple endocrine neoplasia type 2). They have been shown to have beneficial extraglycemic effects such as reduction in cardiovascular events and reduction in nephropathy progression. They also have early data on reduction in nonalcoholic steatohepatitis (NASH) progression and may provide some cognitive protection.

Dual GLP-1RA/GIP RA: This is a new medication at the time of this edition. Tirzepatide is a dual receptor agonist for both GLP-1/GIP. This medication is provided once weekly by subcutaneous injection. It is biochemically more like a GIP, but it has GLP-1RA-like effects. Patients have similar GI side effects and warnings like the GLP-1RA but have even greater weight loss. There are no currently known benefits from cardiovascular or extraglycemic benefits, and no long-term safety yet. This is a branded and expensive medication.

SGLT-2 inhibitors: This class of medications function in the kidneys by reducing renal tubular glucose reabsorption, producing a reduction in blood glucose without stimulating insulin release. SGLT-2 inhibitors also affect tubuloglomerular feedback, which may be important for its extraglycemic effects. This class is unique in that they do not require a normal functioning pancreas to implement glucose lowering. They are once-daily tablets and will impact both the fasting and postprandial glucose, but they are not as effective as the GLP-1RA in glucose lowering. They are weight neutral. They do not typically cause hypoglycemia in most people. Their most common side effects are UTIs and genital yeast infections. Their glucose-lowering effect is impacted by renal function and should not be relied on for glycemic control at an eGFR < 45 mL/min. But they will still provide cardiac and kidney benefits all the way down to an eGFR of 25 mL/min. These medications are branded and expensive. They have been shown to have extraglycemic effects such as reduction in cardiovascular events, reduction in nephropathy progression, and reduction in heart failure hospitalizations. Certain SGLT-2 inhibitors have been approved for use in patients with heart failure independent of having diabetes. Their use for kidney protection and heart failure is not limited by renal function.

Alpha glucosidase inhibitors: These work to delay the absorption of carbohydrates from the small intestine. Their mechanism of action is to competitively inhibit enzymes that convert complex nonabsorbable carbohydrates into simple absorbable carbohydrates. They are short acting and are only taken with meals. Therefore, their effect is only on postprandial glucose levels. Their most common side effects are lower GI related, including flatulence and diarrhea. They have a relatively low risk of hypoglycemia; however, due to their mechanism of action, if a person does experience hypoglycemia on these medications, they must be treated with pure glucose. Some people use these only for high-carb meals.

Thiazolidinediones (TZDs): TZDs are insulin sensitizers that act to enhance insulin action and increase insulin sensitivity. TZDs also promote hormonal effects that decrease hepatic gluconeogenesis and increase insulin-dependent glucose uptake in muscle and fat. These are inexpensive tablets taken once daily. They work very slowly, taking up to 16 weeks to get a maximal glucose-lowering effect. They primarily impact the fasting glucose. Only one TZD, pioglitazone, is currently available in the United States without special exceptions. Another TZD was removed from use due to its association with adverse cardiovascular events. This led to the Food and Drug Administration (FDA) developing a "Guidance for Industry" in 2008, requiring that all future antidiabetic medications provide evidence that they do not increase cardiovascular risk. Pioglitazone can cause weight gain and fluid retention and has been associated with a dose-dependent exacerbation of heart failure. TZDs have been associated with increased bone loss resulting in non–weight bearing bone fractures. This is more likely to occur in women. There have been mixed studies regarding TZD use and an increased risk of bladder cancer. Because of this there is a recommendation to use the lowest effective dose, and limit use to no longer than 5 years. Pioglitazone also reduces triglycerides and has been shown to prevent the progression of NASH.

Colesevelam: This medication was developed to treat hypercholesterolemia but was found to also lower glucose. While the mechanism of its glycemic effect is not completely understood it is believed that colesevelam increases incretin-based insulin secretion but does not affect gluconeogenesis.[6] Side effects from colesevelam are mostly GI-related, including nausea, abdominal pain, bloating, increased flatulence, and constipation or diarrhea. It is moderately expensive. This medication does have the benefit of lowering both glucose and LDL (low-density lipoprotein) cholesterol.

Bromocriptine: This is a medication used less often for the treatment of diabetes. It is newer medication that works via the hunger centers to reduce glucose. Its effect is mild with a mean 0.27% decrease in HbA1c. It is branded and expensive. First-dose hypotension is one of the major concerns with this medication.

Amylin mimetics: Pramlintide is an amylin mimetic. This medication is an incretin agent that is given by subcutaneous injection before each meal. It replicates the action of amylin—a hormone that is endogenously secreted with insulin. In people with type 1 diabetes they are deficient in amylin and in type 2 diabetes resistant to amylin. When provided pharmacologically, it reduces postprandial glucose and reduces the amount of insulin needed at that meal. It is also associated with some weight loss. As an incretin it does have similar GI side effects including nausea, loss of appetite, and vomiting. It is also associated with higher rates of hypoglycemia when it is administered with insulin.

3. When selecting combination therapies for people with type 2 diabetes it is best to think about the pathophysiology of the condition and select treatments that will address different aspects of the pathophysiology.

For example a commonly used combination is metformin (which suppresses hepatic glucose production and a sulfonylurea which stimulates increase in insulin release. This combination could be modified by switching the SU for a DPP-4 inhibitor. The DPP-4 inhibitor will focus on postprandial glucose and has no associated weight gain or increased risk of hypoglycemia.

Another great combination is the use of the GLP-1RA (works on suppressing glucagon and glucose dependent insulin secretion) and the SGLT2- inhibitors (change renal threshold for glucose urinary excretion). These are agents both lower fasting and postprandial glucose without a significant increase in hypoglycemia. This combination can provide significant A1c reduction and weight loss. They are both branded classes of medication so cost and coverage would need to be considered.

Case Summary and Closing Points

There are many classes of medications available to treat diabetes. While not all medications get used equally, a good working knowledge of these medications is recommended to allow the clinician to most effectively individualize treatment for patients with type 2 diabetes. In general, when choosing a medication, consider the following, (1) what glucose value are you trying to address (fasting vs postprandial), (2) how much power do you need, (3) what is the cost of this medication, and (4) which medications best match the patient's preferences.

References

1. Kalyani RR. Glucose-lowering drugs to reduce cardiovascular risk in type 2 diabetes. *N Engl J Med.* 2021;384(13):1248-1260. doi:10.1056/NEJMcp2000280
2. Young CF, Dugan J, Pfotenhauer K, Shubrook JH. Pharmacologic management of type 2 diabetes. Part 1. *Prim Care Rep.* 2016;22(10):117-127.
3. Young CF, Dugan J, Pfotenhauer K, Shubrook JH. Pharmacologic management of type 2 diabetes. Part 2. *Prim Care Rep.* 2016;22(11)129-139.
4. Ting RZW, Szeto CC, Chan MHM, Ma KK, Chow KM. Risk factors of vitamin B12 deficiency in patients receiving metformin. *Arch Intern Med.* 2006;166(18):1975-1979. doi:10.1001/archinte.166.18.1975.
5. Metformin Package Insert: Approved 1995. Accesses December 28, 2022. https://www.accessdata.fda.gov/drugsatfda_docs/label/2017/020357s037s039,021202s021s023lbl.pdf
6. Beysen C, Murphy EJ, Deines K, et al. Effect of bile acid sequestrants on glucose metabolism, hepatic de novo lipogenesis, and cholesterol and bile acid kinetics in type 2 diabetes: a randomised controlled study. *Diabetologia.* 2012;55:432-442. doi:10.1007/s00125-011-2382-3

Case 4.   Extraglycemic Effects of Medications

"You mean this treats my whole body?"

A 48-year-old man with type 2 diabetes for 6 years presents with questions about his diabetes management. He recently heard that some diabetes medications can reduce his risk for heart disease and kidney disease. He wants to know if he should be on one of these since he was first diagnosed with diabetes when he had a heart attack.

Med HX: type 2 diabetes mellitus (DM), hypertension, ASCVD s/p stent placement left circumflex, dyslipidemia

Medications: metformin 1000 mg po bid, empagliflozin 25 mg daily, dulaglutide 1.5 mg weekly, lisinopril 40 daily, atorvastatin 80 mg daily, carvedilol 12.5 mg bid, acetylsalicylic acid (ASA) 325 mg daily.

Allergies: none

Family Medical History: type 2 diabetes in both parents, father died at 56 with myocardial infarction (MI), mom alive at 70 but has had a cerebrovascular accident (CVA)

Social History: no tobacco, no alcohol, and no recreational drug use. He has a room-mate but is single and not in a current relationship. He is employed as an accountant. He follows a Mediterranean diet, and tries to walk at least 3 times per week.

Physical Exam: Ht. 5′8″, Wt. 198 lb, BMI 30, T 98.2, P 78, R 12, BP 102/68

GEN: in no distress

HEENT: normal including thyroid exam

CV: rate and rhythm regular, peripheral pulses present

RESP: normal

Diabetes foot exam: normal pulses, no calluses, or skin breakdown, normal sensation to monofilament, no edema

His labs are normal and his HbA1c is 6.6%, which has been stable for about a year.

 CASE QUESTIONS

1. What diabetes medications have extraglycemic benefits?
2. What medications have FDA indications other than diabetes?
3. How would you change his treatment plan?

 ANSWERS AND EXPLANATIONS

1. Traditionally, clinicians' major concern with diabetes medications was their effect on blood sugar control. Now, there is evidence that many diabetes medications can positively impact other health conditions and prevent certain diabetes-related complications. The American Association of Clinical Endocrinologists has included a review of each of the diabetes medications as part of its guidance for the treatment of hyperglycemia.[1]

Classes of medications that have been shown to reduce weight:	SGLT-2i, GLP-1RA, pramlintide, dual GLP-1/GIP RA
Classes of medications that lower BP:	SGLT-2 inhibitor, GLP-1RA
Class of medication that lower cholesterol:	colesevelam
Classes of medications that have been shown to reduce coronary events:	SGLT-2 inhibitor, GLP-1RA
Classes of medications that have been shown to reduce ischemic stroke:	GLP-1RA, TZD
Classes of medication that have been shown to reduce progression of NASH:	TZDs, GLP-1RA (Figure 4.1)

PROFILES OF ANTIDIABETIC MEDICATIONS

	MET	GLP1-RA	SGLT2i	DPP4i	AGi	TZD (moderate dose)	SU / GLN	COLSVL	BCR-QR	INSULIN	PRAML
HYPO	Neutral	Neutral	Neutral	Neutral	Neutral	Neutral	Moderate/Severe (SU) / Mild (GLN)	Neutral	Neutral	Moderate to Severe	Neutral
WEIGHT	Slight Loss	Loss	Loss	Neutral	Neutral	Gain	Gain	Neutral	Neutral	Gain	Loss
RENAL / GU	Contraindicated if eGFR <30 mL/min/1.73 m²	Exenatide Not Indicated CrCl <30 / Possible Benefit of Liraglutide	Not indicated for eGFR <45 mL/min/1.73 m² / Genital Mycotic Infections / Possible CKD Benefit	Dose Adjustment Necessary (Except Linagliptin) / Effective in Reducing Albuminuria	Neutral	Neutral	More Hypo Risk	Neutral	Neutral	More Hypo Risk	Neutral
GI Sx	Moderate	Moderate	Neutral	Neutral	Moderate	Neutral	Neutral	Mild	Moderate	Neutral	Moderate
CHF	Neutral	See #1	See #2		Neutral	Moderate	Neutral	Neutral	Neutral	CHF Risk	Neutral
CARDIAC — ASCVD	Neutral			See #3	Neutral	May Reduce Stroke Risk	Possible ASCVD Risk	Benefit	Safe	Neutral	Neutral
BONE	Neutral	Neutral	Neutral	Neutral	Neutral	Moderate Fracture Risk	Neutral	Neutral	Neutral	Neutral	Neutral
KETOACIDOSIS	Neutral	Neutral	DKA Can Occur in Various Stress Settings	Neutral	Neutral	Neutral	Neutral	Neutral	Neutral	Neutral	Neutral

■ Few adverse events or possible benefits
■ Use with caution
■ Likelihood of adverse effects

1. Liraglutide—FDA approved for prevention of MACE events.
2. Empagliflozin—FDA approved to reduce CV mortality. Canagliflozin—FDA approved to reduce MACE events.
3. Possible increased hospitalizations for heart failure with alogliptin and saxagliptin.

FIGURE 4.1. **AACE hyperglycemic algorithm—profiles of antihyperglycemic medication.** (Used with permission from AACE.)

2. The FDA required all new diabetes medications from 2008 onward to show not only efficacy in reducing glucose but also evidence from cardiovascular outcome trials that the agent did not cause an increase in vascular events.[2] The findings from these trials showed additional benefits beyond glucose control and no excess cardiovascular risk. The data are described below, and there are excellent reviews on the topic.[3-6]

FDA-approved (2022) nonglycemic indications of antidiabetes medications:
To reduce cardiovascular risk in people with established CVD
To reduce cardiovascular risk in people with risk factors for ASCVD
To reduce risk of hospitalization for heart failure
To reduce the risk of cardiovascular death in adults with heart failure
To reduce risk of diabetic kidney disease (Tables 4.4 and 4.5)

1. This is a relatively young patient with well-controlled type 2 DM and known CVD. Based on ADA and American College of Cardiology (ACC) guidelines he would benefit from a treatment regimen proven to reduce future cardiovascular risk. This recommendation is independent of his current degree of glycemic levels. Agents that should be considered are the GLP-1RAs (dulaglutide, liraglutide, semaglutide weekly) and the SGLT-2 inhibitors (canagliflozin, empagliflozin) (Table 4.6).

TABLE 4.4   GLP-1RA and Extraglycemic Effects

Medication	MACE	Nephropathy	Heart Failure	Weight
Lixisenatide	Neutral			Decreased
Exenatide (bid)	Not studied			Decreased
Liraglutide	Decreased	Decreased		Decreased
Exenatide weekly	Neutral			Decreased
Dulaglutide	Decreased	Decreased		Decreased
Semaglutide weekly	Decreased	Decreased		Decreased
Semaglutide oral	Neutral	Not studied		Decreased

MACE, major adverse cardiovascular events

TABLE 4.5   SGLT-2 Inhibitors and Extraglycemic Effects

Medication	Major Cardiovascular Events	Nephropathy	Heart Failure	Weight
Canagliflozin	Decreased	Decreased	Decreased	Decreased
Dapagliflozin	Neutral	Decreased	Decreased	Decreased
Empagliflozin	Decreased	Decreased	Decreased	Decreased
Ertugliflozin	Neutral	Neutral	Decreased	Decreased

TABLE 4.6   Clinical Trials Showing Cardiovascular Benefit of Glucose-Lowering Agents in Patients With Type 2 Diabetes[a]

Class and Drug With CVD Benefit in Specific Study Populations	Clinical Trial	Primary and Secondary Outcomes With Significant Risk Reductions	
		Major Adverse Cardiovascular Events[b]	Hospitalization for Heart Failure
Established CVD			
GLP-1 receptor agonists			
Liraglutide	Liraglutide Effect and Action in Diabetes: Evaluation of Cardiovascular Outcome Results (LEADER)[7]	Primary outcome[c]	
Semaglutide[d]	Trial to Evaluate Cardiovascular and Other Long-term Outcomes With Semaglutide in Subjects With Type 2 Diabetes (SUSTAIN-6)[8]	Primary outcome[c]	
Dulaglutide	Researching Cardiovascular Events With a Weekly Incretin in Diabetes (REWIND)[9]	Primary outcome[c]	
SGLT-2 inhibitors			
Empagliflozin	Empagliflozin Cardiovascular Outcome Event Trial in Type 2 Diabetes Mellitus Patients (EMPA-REG)[10]	Primary outcome[c]	Secondary outcome
Canagliflozin	Canagliflozin Cardiovascular Assessment Study (CANVAS)[11]	Primary outcome[c]	Secondary outcome
Dapagliflozin	Dapagliflozin Effect on Cardiovascular Events—Thrombolysis in Myocardial Infarction 58 (DECLARE-TIMI 58)[12]		Primary outcome[c,e]

TABLE 4.6   Clinical Trials Showing Cardiovascular Benefit of Glucose-Lowering Agents in Patients With Type 2 Diabetes[a]   (Continued)

Class and Drug With CVD Benefit in Specific Study Populations	Clinical Trial	Primary and Secondary Outcomes With Significant Risk Reductions	
		Major Adverse Cardiovascular Events[b]	Hospitalization for Heart Failure
Ertugliflozin	Evaluation of Ertugliflozin Efficacy and Safety Cardiovascular Outcomes Trial (VERTIS CV)[13]		Secondary outcome
Multiple CVD Risk Factors			
GLP-1 receptor agonist, dulaglutide	Researching Cardiovascular Events With a Weekly Incretin in Diabetes (REWIND)[9]	Primary outcome[c]	
SGLT-2 inhibitor, dapagliflozin	Dapagliflozin Effect on Cardiovascular Events–Thrombolysis in Myocardial Infarction 58 (DECLARE-TIMI 58)[12]		Primary outcome[c,e]
Heart Failure With Rejection Fraction[f]			
SGLT-2 inhibitors			
Dapagliflozin	Dapagliflozin and Prevention of Adverse Outcomes in Heart Failure (DAPA-HF)[14,c]		Primary outcome[c,e]
Empagliflozin	Empagliflozin Outcome Trial in Patients with Chronic Heart Failure and a Reduced Ejection Fraction (EMPEROR-Reduced)[15]		Primary outcome[e]

(Continued)

TABLE 4.6   Clinical Trials Showing Cardiovascular Benefit of Glucose-Lowering Agents in Patients With Type 2 Diabetes[a]   (Continued)

Class and Drug With CVD Benefit in Specific Study Populations	Clinical Trial	Primary and Secondary Outcomes With Significant Risk Reductions	
		Major Adverse Cardiovascular Events[b]	Hospitalization for Heart Failure
Albuminuric Chronic Kidney Disease[g]			
SGLT-2 inhibitors			
Canagliflozin	Canagliflozin and Renal Events in Diabetes with Established Nephropathy Clinical Evaluation (CREDENCE)[16]	Secondary outcome	Secondary outcome[c]
Dapagliflozin	Dapagliflozin and Prevention of Adverse Outcomes in Chronic Kidney Disease (DAPA-CKD)[17]	Secondary outcome	Secondary outcome

CVD, cardiovascular disease.

What you will find in the Kalyani RR Table NEJM

Used with permission from Kalyani RR. Glucose-lowering drugs to reduce cardiovascular risk in type 2 diabetes. *N Engl J Med (NEJM)*. 2021;384(13):1248-1260. Massachusetts Medical Society.

[a]Some agents are beneficial in reducing the risk of worsening nephropathy as a secondary outcome, but only cardiovascular benefits are shown. GLP-1 denotes glucagon-like peptide-1 and SGLT-2, sodium-glucose transporter type 2.

[b]Major adverse cardiovascular events included nonfatal myocardial infarction, nonfatal stroke, and death from cardiovascular disease (CVD).

[c]These agents have a label indication from the Food and Drug Administration indicating a reduction in this cardiovascular outcome in the specific population of patients listed with type 2 diabetes.

[d]Only the injectable version of semaglutide has demonstrated CVD benefit.

[e]The primary outcome included hospitalization for heart failure and cardiovascular death (and, in DAPA-HF [Dapagliflozin and Prevention of Adverse Outcomes in Heart Failure], an urgent visit for heart failure).

[f]Ongoing placebo-controlled trials are investigating the use of dapagliflozin (ClinicalTrials.gov number, NCT03619213) and empagliflozin (ClinicalTrials.gov number, NCT03057951) in the treatment of heart failure with preserved ejection fraction.

[g]Ongoing placebo-controlled trials are investigating the use of empagliflozin (Clinicaltrials.gov number, NCT03594110) and semaglutide (Clinicaltrials.gov number, NCT03819153) in patients with chronic kidney disease.

Case Summary and Closing Points

This is an exciting time to be treating people with diabetes. For decades, clinicians were limited to lowering glucose levels. Research studies revealed, though, that glucose control can reduce microvascular complications (nephropathy, neuropathy, retinopathy). In fact, newer diabetes medications can reduce cardiovascular events and improve CKD and heart failure. Emerging research is showing that some of the newer medications may improve NASH and even cognition. Be sure to share with patients that new medications can have multiple positive benefits. The challenge to keep up with the data is constant. Resources like the ADA Standards of Care for people with diabetes and the Abridged Standards of Care for primary care are published annually and are great resources for the busy clinician.

References

1. American Association of Clinical Endocrinologists (AACE). Comprehensive Type 2 Diabetes Management Algorithm (2020)—EXECUTIVE SUMMARY. 2019. Accessed December 28, 2022. https://pro.aace.com/pdfs/diabetes/AACE_2019_Diabetes_Algorithm_03.2021.pdf
2. Food and Drug Administration. *Guidance for Industry: Diabetes Mellitus—Evaluating Cardiovascular Risk in New Antidiabetic Therapies to Treat Type 2 Diabetes.* 2008. Accessed December 28, 2022. https://www.fda.gov/media/71297/download
3. Kalyani RR. Glucose-lowering drugs to reduce cardiovascular risk in type 2 diabetes. *N Engl J Med.* 2021;384(13):1248-1260. doi:10.1056/NEJMcp2000280
4. McGuire DK, Shih WJ, Cosentino F, et al. Association of SGLT2 inhibitors with cardiovascular and kidney outcomes in patients with type 2 diabetes: a meta-analysis. *JAMA Cardiol.* 2021;6(2):148-158.
5. Gotfried R. How to use type 2 diabetes meds to lower CV disease risk. *J Fam Pract.* 2019;68(9):494;498;500;504.
6. Young CF, Dugan J, Pfotenhauer K, Shubrook JH. Pharmacologic management of type 2 diabetes. Part 2. *Prim Care Rep.* 2016;22(10):117-127.
7. Marso SP, Daniels GH, Brown-Frandsen K, et al. Liraglutide and cardiovascular outcomes in type 2 diabetes. *N Engl J Med.* 2016;375:311-322.
8. Marso SP, Bain SC, Consoli A, et al. Semaglutide and cardiovascular outcomes in patients with type 2 diabetes. *N Engl J Med.* 2016;375:1834-1844.
9. Gerstein HC, Colhoun HM, Dagenais GR, et al. Dulaglutide and cardiovascular outcomes in type 2 diabetes (REWIND): a double-blind, randomised placebo-controlled trial. *Lancet.* 2019;394:121-130.
10. Zinman B, Wanner C, Lachin JM, et al. Empagliflozin, cardiovascular outcomes, and mortality in type 2 diabetes. *N Engl J Med.* 2015;373:2117-2128.
11. Neal B, Perkovic V, Mahaffey KW, et al. Canagliflozin and cardiovascular and renal events in type 2 diabetes. *N Engl J Med.* 2017;377:644-657.
12. Wiviott SD, Raz I, Bonaca MP, et al. Dapagliflozin and cardiovascular outcomes in type 2 diabetes. *N Engl J Med.* 2019;380:347-357.
13. Cannon CP, Pratley R, Dagogo-Jack S, et al. Cardiovascular outcomes with ertugliflozin in type 2 diabetes. *N Engl J Med.* 2020;383:1425-1435.
14. McMurray JJV, Solomon SD, Inzucchi SE, et al. Dapagliflozin in patients with heart failure and reduced ejection fraction. *N Engl J Med.* 2019;381:1995-2008.
15. Packer M, Anker SD, Butler J, et al. Cardiovascular and renal outcomes with empagliflozin in heart failure. *N Engl J Med.* 2020;383:1413-1424.
16. Perkovic V, Jardine MJ, Neal B, et al. Canagliflozin and renal outcomes in type 2 diabetes and nephropathy. *N Engl J Med.* 2019;380:2295-2306.
17. Heerspink HJL, Stefánsson BV, Correa-Rotter R, et al. Dapagliflozin in patients with chronic kidney disease. *N Engl J Med.* 2020;383:1436-1446.

Case 5. Best Practices in Starting Insulin

"You mean I need insulin?"

A 74-year-old man presents for a recheck on his diabetes. He has had type 2 diabetes for 24 years. He worked hard to take care of himself both in terms of eating well and staying active. This has gotten more difficult over the years. He has developed bad feet and knees and this has really changed his activity level. He had been very diligent about checking his blood sugars and previously used a continuous glucose monitor (CGM), which he had found to be really helpful. In the past, it had enabled him to see how certain foods affected his glucose and then make changes. Over the past year, he has struggled more with his diet. He used to come to his appointments regularly but has not been seen for a year. His wife has become more dependent on him for care and it has been difficult for him to get out of the house.

Med HX: type 2 DM, hypertension, benign prostatic hyperplasia, dyslipidemia, knee osteoarthritis (OA)

Medications: metformin 1000 mg bid, empagliflozin 25 mg daily, oral semaglutide 14 mg daily, acarbose 25 mg tid qac, lisinopril HCT 20/25 daily, atorvastatin 80 mg daily, meloxicam 15 mg daily

Allergies: sulfa—rash

Family Medical History: noncontributory

Social History: no tobacco, no alcohol, and no recreational drug use. He lives with his spouse for 50 years. He used to get out more, but he is the full-time caregiver for his spouse who has dementia. He has two adult children, and four grandchildren who he sees on a regular basis.

Physical Exam: Ht. 6′0″, Wt. 202 lb, BMI 27.4, T 98.2, P 78, R 12, BP 112/70

GEN: in no distress

HEENT: normal including thyroid exam

CV: SEM at base of heart parasternal, rate and rhythm regular, peripheral pulses present

RESP: normal

Extremities: no edema, diabetes foot exam reveals loss of sensation to light touch and vibration in multiple toes. Bunions noted and calluses present at the medial aspect of both first metatarsal-phalangeal joints.

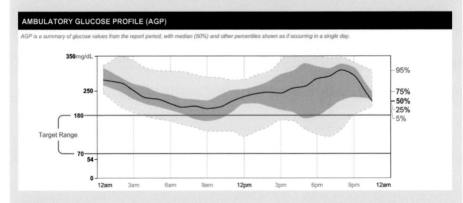

AMBULATORY GLUCOSE PROFILE (AGP)

AGP is a summary of glucose values from the report period, with median (50%) and other percentiles shown as if occurring in a single day.

Labs:

Comprehensive Metabolic Panel	Value	Reference Range
Sodium	141	136-145 mmol/L
Potassium, serum	3.8	3.5-5.3 mmol/L

Comprehensive Metabolic Panel	Value	Reference Range
Chloride, serum	99	98-110 mmol/L
Carbon dioxide (CO_2)	26	19-30 mmol/L
Urea nitrogen, blood (BUN)	15	7-25 mg/dL
Creatinine, serum	1.2	0.5-1.10 mg/dL
eGFR	78	>60 mL/min/1.73 m²
Glucose, serum	182	65-99 mg/dL
Calcium, serum	9.9	8.6-10.2 mg/dL
Protein, total	7.1	6.1-8.1 g/dL
Albumin	4.3	3.6-4.1 g/dL
Globulin	2.8	1.9-3.7 g/dL
AST (SGOT)	20	10-35 U/L
ALT (SGPT)	22	6-29 U/L
Bilirubin, total	0.7	0.2-1.2 mg/dL
Alkaline phosphatase	100	33-115 U/L

Lipid Panel	Value	Reference Range
Cholesterol, total	130	125-200 mg/dL
Triglycerides	154	<150 mg/dL
LDL (calculated)	60	<130 mg/dL
HDL cholesterol	42	>40 mg/dL men; >50 women
Non-HDL cholesterol	78	<130

Other Labs	Value	Reference Range
HbA1c	10.2%	<5.7% (normal)
Urine albumin/creatinine ratio (UACr)	88 mg/G	<30 mg/G

 CASE QUESTIONS

1. Is it typical for a patient like this to need insulin?
2. What lifestyle changes may be helpful?
3. What medications would you add? Would you stop any of his current medications?
4. If you choose insulin, how would you start it and adjust the dose?

 ANSWERS AND EXPLANATIONS

1. Type 2 diabetes is a progressive condition characterized by declining beta cell function over time. As discussed above, beta cell function may be preserved in some people, but the reality is most patients will need insulin to manage their diabetes after about 10 years of diabetes duration.

As this case exemplifies, this should not be seen as a failure to manage diabetes but rather as a common problem arising from this chronic disease. In fact, this patient should be congratulated for managing his diabetes for 20 years without needing insulin. Celebrating the things that have worked for him reinforces the value of these self-care behaviors to minimize the impact that diabetes has on his health.

He is currently taking four glucose-lowering medications and his A1c is above 10%. It is unlikely, even using an age-based relaxed goal of 8%, that he will achieve this without the addition of insulin.

2. He has had success with lifestyle change in the past. It is important to help him get back to a lower carbohydrate dietary plan and find a way he can be more physically active without pain. Options such as a stationary bike, exercising in a pool, and a meal plan such as *Weight Watchers* or *Slimfast* could help. Of course, he will need help balancing between taking care of his wife and finding time to do self-care. A home health aide or a senior center that can provide daycare or even full-time care for his wife also may be options. Asking his children for help could be a consideration as well.

3. Recognizing that his A1c is at least 2% above goal despite using four antidiabetic medications, insulin is his best option. It is one of the most potent medications, and it can help him reduce his other medication burden. Adding other oral medications is unlikely to provide much benefit.

Reviewing his CGM download, he appears to be hyperglycemic all the time and he is not having any hypoglycemia. Having CGM data makes this decision rather straightforward. With persistent hyperglycemia throughout the day, it is prudent to "fix the fasting first." This can be completed with the use of a basal insulin.

In terms of reducing his medication burden there are a couple of options. You may choose not to reduce medications if the A1c is above 10% unless the person is having hypoglycemic episodes. However, the acarbose is the least likely to provide much benefit and it is 3 times a day so you could consider stopping this. One option is to stop metformin, especially if he can get his BMI to below 25 kg/m^2. This is a nice way to encourage lifestyle change as a replacement for some medications.

4. There is ample evidence that too often insulin is not started at an adequate dose or titrated enough to provide benefit.[1] In fact, multiple studies have shown only about one-third of people who start insulin are at goal at 3 months.[2,3] Those who are not at goal at 3 months are also not likely to be at goal by 1 year.[2] Therefore, it is important to focus on getting to goal within the first 3 months of starting insulin.

Key errors to avoid when starting basal insulin:

1. Not using an adequate starting dose
2. Not teaching the patient to titrate to a fasting glucose goal
3. Not having early follow-up appointments
4. Not teaching the patient how to inject insulin properly

To help him gain confidence in the use of insulin, it is important to pick a starting dose that will clearly make a difference in his fasting glucose. The best way to achieve this is to use a weight-based dose. Starting with 0.2 U/kg to 0.3 U/kg/d will be both safe and effective in people with type 2 diabetes.

For this patient 20 to 30 U/d is a good starting dose. Since injections are a new skill for him, it is important that he be taught how to safely administer insulin. This can be done during the office visit, administering the first injection in the office. If this is not an option, he can schedule an appointment with a diabetes care and education specialist or a PharmD who can help teach him how to do the injections. Ideally, he would use an insulin pen as most people find using insulin pens is much simpler than using vials and syringes.

Any of the basal insulin options are acceptable. At first, once-daily dosing is sufficient. There are many approaches to self-titration. They can be equally effective. The key is to empower the patient to titrate their dosage at home. It is also important for the provider to be willing to enable the patient to self-titrate their dosage.

Three common basal insulin titration strategies:
These regimens are utilized to help the patient achieve a goal fasting glucose, typically 120 mg/dL. The patient is instructed to add a specific amount to their basal dose at a defined interval. They are also given instructions about how to reduce their dose should their fasting drop too low.

1. Add 1 unit to the dose every day
2. Add 3 to 5 units 2 times a week
3. Add 5 to 7 units once weekly

Each of these insulin titration algorithms are utilized to one of these stopping points:

1. Agreed fasting glucose have been achieved
2. Patient is experiencing hypoglycemia
3. Total basal dose has reached 0.5 U/kg/d

These endpoints are important as they help protect the patient from excessive dosing and hypoglycemia.

Self-titration requires the patient to be an active participant in their medical care. To be successful they need to engage in self-monitoring, and to take a role in their insulin dosing. By creating a treatment plan the patient has a role in managing, you help to strengthen your partnership. A self-titration approach also provides you and the patient a framework to set your agenda for their next visit, to assess their results.

This is also a great time to let the patient know that at that visit you could review reducing or stopping some of their other medications. If this patient was on a sulfonylurea or meglitinide, these would be the first medications to remove. He is not on any medication that typically causes hypoglycemia, so you have the luxury to review his medications with him and decide which medications he may prefer to stop.

At your next visit, he mentions that while metformin has helped control his blood sugars, he has found that even after using it for many years it still bothers his stomach. Often, he must eat to limit the side effect, at times eating just so he can take the medication. Considering that metformin's effect primarily is on the fasting glucose, which is what his basal insulin is now addressing, it is reasonable to stop this. Since he will be modifying his diet to reduce his carbohydrate intake, acarbose will likely have less of an impact in controlling his postprandial glucose.

He can discontinue this as well. By introducing a single basal insulin dose, he can eliminate two oral medications and five pills a day.

An important caveat: be careful to not use too much basal insulin. Doses above 0.5 U/kg/d have been shown to cause more problems with hypoglycemia and weight gain without meaningful benefit in glucose reduction.[4]

Case Summary and Closing Points

Starting insulin is a really big deal for most patients. Having clear guidelines as to when insulin is the optimal treatment and outlining what insulin will do for the patient can make the adjustment easier. Since this is a big step for patients, make sure it is successful, that is, make a positive difference for the patient. Start with a weight-based dose. Then, let the patient titrate the dose. Have a clear stopping point at which you and the patient can reassess the treatment plan. When done well, insulin can often simplify a patient's regimen and allow them to feel in control again. Done poorly, insulin can really frustrate your patients.

References

1. Khunti K, Nikolajsen A, Thorsted BL, Andersen M, Davies MJ, Paul SK. Clinical inertia with regard to intensifying therapy in people with type 2 diabetes treated with basal insulin. *Diabetes Obes Metab.* 2016;18(4):401-409.
2. Blonde L, Meneghini L, Peng XV, et al. Probability of achieving glycemic control with basal insulin in patients with type 2 diabetes in real-world practice in the USA. *Diabetes Ther.* 2018;9(3):1347-1358.
3. The diabetes unmet need with basal insulin evaluation (DUNE) study in type 2 diabetes. *Diabetes Obes Metabol.* 2019;21(6):1429-1436.
4. Reid T, Gao L, Gill J, et al. How much is too much? Outcomes in patients using high dose insulin glargine. *Int J Clin Pract.* 2016;70(1):56-65.

Case 6. Effective Correction Insulin

"They put me on sliding scale"

A 53-year-old woman returns to the office 1 month after being hospitalized for cholecystitis. She is feeling much better since her gallbladder was removed. During her stay the hospitalist raised her basal insulin dose and added a short-acting insulin sliding scale for meals. She is not sure this insulin has helped. Her fingersticks always seem to be high after she eats; however, since being discharged from the hospital she has noticed she is having lows if she does not eat.

Glucose log:

	Monday	Tuesday	Wednesday	Thursday	Friday	Saturday	Sunday
Prebreakfast	104	98	158	107	156	109	90
Prelunch		168		60			
Predinner		224	220	249	223		56
Bedtime							
Notes				Missed lunch			Missed lunch

Med HX: type 2 DM, hypertension, dyslipidemia, mild intermittent asthma, cholecystectomy

Medications: metformin 1000 mg po bid, insulin glargine 45 units daily, insulin aspart by sliding scale, lisinopril HCT 20/25 daily, atorvastatin 80 mg daily

Allergies: Sulfa—rash

Family Medical History: type 2 DM in both parents, lung cancer in father, asthma in sister

Social History: no tobacco, no alcohol, and no recreational drug use

Physical Exam: Ht. 5′7″, Wt. 202 lb, BMI 31.6, T 98.2, P 78, R 12, BP 136/74

GEN: in no distress

HEENT: normal including thyroid exam

CV: rate and rhythm regular, peripheral pulses present

RESP: normal

Abdomen: scars appropriate to surgical history, no tenderness, and no masses appreciated

Extremities: no edema, diabetes foot exam normal

Patient's correction scale is as follows:

Check glucose after meals: if glucose is:

<150	No Insulin
151-200	1 unit
201-250	2 units
251-300	3 units
301-350	4 units
>350	5 units

CASE QUESTIONS

1. What is a sliding scale and how does it differ from a correction scale?
2. What would you recommend in terms of medication adjustments?
3. How would you start a mealtime insulin dose with a correction scale?

ANSWERS AND EXPLANATIONS

1. Sliding scale insulin is a method of insulin dosing typically started in a hospital setting when a person is hyperglycemic but their response to insulin is unknown. It involves administration of a short-acting insulin on a schedule, not necessarily in conjunction with meals. This can be an effective way to prevent excessive hyperglycemia while the patient is ill.

Typically, a formula based on random fingersticks is utilized to determine one's dose. Many clinicians often use the same formula for all their patients regardless of their diabetes type, the severity of their illness, or their need for hospitalization. This is not a prudent approach to insulin management. A single sliding scale for all patients is likely to overdose people with type 1 diabetes and underdose people with type 2 diabetes.

The best practice for using a sliding scale is to use the information gained from the amount of short-acting insulin needed during the first 24 hours and incorporate that amount of insulin into scheduled mealtime insulin doses. While a sliding scale may be necessary in the first 24 hours in the hospital, we can use the information gained to make a specific correction scale that is more likely to help the patient.

The correction scale takes patient factors into account: type of diabetes, weight, insulin sensitivity, basal insulin dose, and sometimes their response to insulin. The patient has type 2 diabetes, is obese, and is already on 45 units of basal insulin. The process for calculating the correction scale in this patient is outlined below.

2. This patient is on metformin and basal insulin. There are no specific treatments to address postprandial hyperglycemia and she is running high after meals. The basal insulin seems to be doing the job to control the fasting glucose, but she has postprandial hyperglycemia, and she will likely need mealtime insulin.

   Increasing the basal insulin is not a good option. This may lower glucose readings around the clock so it may slightly lower the postmeal reading, but it will likely start causing hypoglycemia overnight and during the day if the patient is physically active or has a smaller than normal meal.

   Going back to an earlier case—when the basal insulin dose is above 0.5 U/kg and certainly when it is above 0.7 U/kg the patient is probably on too much basal insulin,[4] and they are at higher risk for hypoglycemia and other insulin excess side effects (fluid retention, increased hunger, and weight gain).

3. There are some assumptions you can use in dosing insulin in type 2 diabetes. Typically, the basal insulin dose will be 50% of total daily insulin needs. She is getting 45 units for her basal needs so she will probably need about that much insulin to cover her meals. While every meal is slightly different most people with type 2 diabetes do not need to carb count to dose insulin. She will probably need about 15 units per meal for 3 meals.

   One option at this point is to start with 10 units with each meal and see how she does—adjusting the meal dose up if needed. This would also allow you to see if you need to reduce her basal insulin once you cover the mealtime more effectively.

   Finally, since you know how much insulin she is taking per day, you can calculate her sensitivity to insulin and provide an individualized correction scale.

To calculate a person's sensitivity to insulin you will need to know:

1. What type of diabetes they have—type 1 (insulin sensitive) or type 2 (insulin resistant)
2. Total daily dose of insulin (add up basal dose plus all of the mealtime doses)

She ended up needing 40 units of basal insulin and 12 units per meal × 3 for a total of 76 U/d. Once you know the total daily dose, use a fixed constant as the nominator:

a. Type 1 diabetes 1800
b. Type 2 diabetes 1500

The patient has type 2 diabetes and takes 76 units total daily dose of insulin.

The sensitivity is then 1500/76 = 19.7 or rounding to 20 units. This means one unit of insulin will drop her glucose by 20 mg/dL. This is helpful as now we can choose a multiplier that is specific to her.

You want to keep her glucose between 100 and 150 mg/dL. To do this, you need to add her "correction insulin dose" to her mealtime dose to get ahead of the hyperglycemia. The correction dose will bring the glucose back into the range, while the mealtime glucose prevents it from climbing with the meal.

Her new scale would look as follows:
1. Basal insulin 30 U/d given at bedtime
2. Mealtime/correction insulin is 10 units per meal plus (this should be given before meals—not after)

<100	−6 units	
100-150	0 unit	
151-170	+1 unit	
171-190	+2 units	
191-210	+3 units	
211-230	+4 units	
231-250	+5 units	
251-270	+6 units	
271-290	+7 units and call	

These calculations may be overwhelming for many patients. One option is to round the insulin sensitivity from 20 to 25 mg/dL and combine to maintain glucose blocks of 50 mg/dL. While this is a little less exact, it will work for many people with type 2 diabetes. In general, if you are going to round, it is better to round up to make sure the person gets a little insulin.

<100	No Insulin Until Eating	
101-150	0 units	
151-200	+2 unit	
201-250	+4 units	
251-300	+6 units	
301-350	+8 units	
>350	+10 units and call	

Case Summary and Closing Points

Adding to basal insulin with mealtime or correction scale insulin can be both complicated and daunting for the clinician and the patient. Whenever possible, use the current insulin dosing for the patient or use a weight-based dose to determine mealtime insulin. Then once you know the total daily dose of insulin needed for a patient, you can calculate their insulin sensitivity to create a correction scale specific to them. This may take some time and focus the first few times you do it, but the process will get easier when done frequently. This method is both more effective and safer than using a sliding scale.

Case 7.	Intensive Insulin Therapy

"This is my short-term plan"

A 68-year-old man presents to you because he needs to have colon surgery and they need him to have better control of his diabetes. He has had diabetes for 6 years and he had good control at first, but his readings started to climb at the beginning of the COVID-19 pandemic and he got frustrated and stopped checking his glucose and getting routine care. His last visit with you was 2 years ago.

He was having some problems with constipation and abdominal pain. They found a mass in the colon, but they are not certain if it is benign or cancerous. The surgery team drew labs on him and wants his A1c to be 7% for him to go to surgery. He wants to figure out what this is and he is anxious to get this done.

Med HX: type 2 DM, hypertension, dyslipidemia, OA knees

Medications: metformin 1000 mg po bid, glipizide 10 mg bid, valsartan 160 mg daily, atorvastatin 10 mg daily

Allergies: none

Family Medical History: diabetes in mother and two brothers, brother had colon cancer (deceased)

Social History: no tobacco, and no recreational drug use; drinks 1 to 2 mixed drinks per day; he lives with his spouse; no regular physical activity

Physical Exam: Ht. 6'2", Wt. 200 lb, BMI 25.7, T 98.2, P 78, R 12, BP: 112/70

GEN: in no distress

HEENT: normal including thyroid exam

CV: normal

RESP: normal

Extremities: normal

Labs:

Comprehensive Metabolic Panel	Value	Reference Range
Sodium	136	136-145 mmol/L
Potassium, serum	3.8	3.5-5.3 mmol/L

Comprehensive Metabolic Panel	Value	Reference Range
Chloride, serum	99	98-110 mmol/L
Carbon dioxide (CO_2)	28	19-30 mmol/L
Urea nitrogen, blood (BUN)	25	7-25 mg/dL
Creatinine, serum	1.3	0.5-1.10 mg/dL
eGFR	52	>60 mL/min/1.73 m²
Glucose, serum	268	65-99 mg/dL
Calcium, serum	9.9	8.6-10.2 mg/dL
Protein, total	6.2	6.1-8.1 g/dL
Albumin	3.9	3.6-4.1 g/dL
Globulin	2.2	1.9-3.7 g/dL
AST (SGOT)	20	10-35 U/L
ALT (SGPT)	22	6-29 U/L
Bilirubin, total	0.7	0.2-1.2 mg/dL
Alkaline phosphatase	100	33-115 U/L

Lipid Panel	Value	Reference Range
Cholesterol, total	210	125-200 mg/dL
Triglycerides	188	<150 mg/dL
LDL (calculated)	140	<130 mg/dL
HDL cholesterol	48	>40 mg/dL men; >50 women
Non-HDL cholesterol	162	<130

Other Labs	Value	Reference Range
HbA1c	9.2%	<5.7% (normal)
Urine albumin/creatinine ratio (UACr)	20 mg/G	<30 mg/G

 CASE QUESTIONS

1. What is the best strategy to help this patient get to surgery?
2. What can we do to speed up the process?
3. What is the long-term plan for him?

 ANSWERS AND EXPLANATIONS

1. He has an immediate need to get control to allow him to have this surgical procedure. In true emergencies—surgeons will often move to surgery immediately. In other cases, improved metabolic control can improve both surgical and recovery outcomes. There is some variability in the preferred glucose control before elective surgeries. Some surgeons will use less than 8.0% and others use less than 7.0%.

This person needs help getting under better glucose control as quickly as possible. The fastest and safest way to get his glucose down to an acceptable level for surgery is insulin. Complete insulin replacement will allow us to get control of his glucose within 1 to 2 weeks if done purposefully.

You have learned the principles of insulin replacement from the earliest cases. Start with a basal insulin and a starting dose of 0.2 to 0.3 U/kg/d. Then, choose one of the patient-driven titration methods (1 U/d, 3-5 units twice weekly, or 5-7 units weekly). Each provides similar amounts per week. Using the twice weekly allows a patient to see the effects with each dose. They will take at least three doses before increasing dosage.

The patient was on metformin and glipizide priorly. If you plan to use the higher dose of insulin, you may consider cutting the dose of glipizide in half or stopping it altogether. Once you have used basal insulin for 1 week, you can start mealtime and correction insulin. This can be done simultaneously. Note, this may be overwhelming for someone who has not taken insulin in the past, so a stepped approach may be more successful at first.

After the first week, the patient should be on a dose of basal insulin that has started to lower the fasting glucose. This will give the patient confidence that he can get his diabetes under control. The next step is to get him on a mealtime insulin. Because time is an important limiting factor, start with 0.1 U/kg/meal at each meal. This is a small enough dose that it is unlikely to cause hypoglycemia and large enough to avoid relying too heavily on basal insulin. With a goal of moving to a full insulin regimen, this would be a good time to stop the sulfonylurea.

Once he is on full insulin replacement (basal and mealtime insulin), he will be in much better control. He will likely need a correction scale, but this can also wait a week or two to let him get used to this regimen.

After 2 weeks, he is taking 33 units of basal insulin and 9 units per meal at every meal. He finds that most of the time his readings are between 100 and 150. He had only one low reading, when he took mealtime insulin but did not actually eat because he took a phone call. He has learned what to eat to keep his glucose from climbing higher with meals. Still, some days, when he has more stress, he runs higher and wants to know what he can do to get it back down.

This is a great time to start a correction scale that he can use when needed. This will be with mealtime insulin—not basal insulin. As mentioned earlier in this chapter, you will need to determine his total daily dose to calculate his sensitivity to insulin.

Basal: 33 units
Mealtime: 9 units × 3= 27 units
Total daily dose: 60 units

Sensitivity: 1500/total daily dose = 25
This means 1 unit of insulin should lower the glucose 25 mg/dL

The goal is to get his glucose between 100 and 150 to help him get to surgery. Give him the option to take correction scale insulin in addition to mealtime insulin before each meal. This can sometimes be given at bedtime, but this dosing should be monitored carefully as it can increase the risk of nocturnal hypoglycemia. His scale:

<150—no additional insulin
150 to 200—2 units
201 to 250—4 units
251 to 300—6 units

This will be used only when he is running higher than normal. Sequentially adding the layers of insulin makes the changes less overwhelming and easier to implement.

2. Based upon his surgeon's requirements, it could take 3 months to get to the goal. You have the patient on the path to success but there are some things that can make this move faster.

   First, send a note to the surgeon that you are working closely with the patient to help them get back under control quickly. You could schedule weekly appointments or telehealth appointments to make sure titrations are occurring and that he is not having any problems (checking glucose, injections, or hypoglycemia).

   This is also a great time to initiate a CGM. The patient will get much more information about glucose levels and the reports could help you and the patient communicate with the surgeon. If you can show a 2-week report with excellent control, the surgeon will likely be more willing to do the surgery earlier than the 3 months it would take to get an HbA1c reduction. Further, good glucose control on a CGM report is probably even safer than relying on a HbA1c that might be missing extreme glucose excursions and hypoglycemia.

3. Once you have helped him reach the management goals for surgery and he is able to have his surgery and recover, he will have lots of choices for diabetes management. It is easier to maintain glycemic targets than to get to them. He may want to stay on basal and bolus insulin therapy as he saw its power and speed. However, he will likely be able to simplify his regimen. This is a great time to discuss the goals the patient has in terms of his treatment so you can do shared decision making and set a regimen that is both effective and fits his life.

Case Summary and Closing Points

When a patient is acutely ill or needs to get under control quickly, a basal and bolus insulin regimen is the quickest way to get there. Once you feel comfortable with weight-based dosing, these steps are pretty easy and will help you and your patient achieve glycemic control quickly. With more intensive insulin regimens, be sure to remind your patients that they will need to monitor their glucose more often. This can be done with multiple daily fingerstick glucose readings or the use of a CGM.

CHAPTER 5 **Hypoglycemia**

Introduction

Hypoglycemia is the rate-limiting factor when treating people with diabetes. Most often hypoglycemia is from diabetes medications. Careful review of the person's daily schedule (meals and activity) can also assist in figuring out the etiology of hypoglycemia. The primary care clinician should be comfortable assessing for hypoglycemia and be able to help patients prevent these episodes. Further, helping the patient address both symptomatic hypoglycemia and severe hypoglycemia are critical skills for people with diabetes.

Case 1.   Reactive Hypoglycemia

"I need to eat, so I do not drop low."

A 43-year-old woman with no diabetes history presents complaining of low blood sugars. Over the last few months, she has been having episodes of feeling shaky, lightheaded, and sweaty after she eats. At first this was uncommon, happening every few weeks but it is occurring more frequently now. Over the last month she has had them several times per week. Usually, they happen 1 to 2 hours after eating. The spells are more likely to occur when she eats rice or pasta. If she eats something sweet when she feels one coming on, she will feel better. She does not have a glucometer, but her friend checked her glucose once during one of the spells and the reading was 64 mg/dL. She is afraid to drive because she is worried that these spells will cause her to pass out.

Med HX: prediabetes, dyslipidemia

Medications: none and no OTC (over-the-counter) supplements or vitamins

Allergies: none

Family Medical History: mother, brother, and maternal grandmother have type 2 diabetes; dad died from a heart attack

Social History: lives with her spouse and two children; works as an administrator; no tobacco use; drinks wine with dinner most nights per week; walks the dog daily morning and evening

Physical Exam: Ht. 5′4″, Wt. 154 lb, BMI 26.4, P 84, R 14, BP 132/74

GEN: in no distress

HEENT: normal including thyroid exam

CV: normal

RESP: normal

Otherwise: normal exam

Labs: all normal except HbA1c 5.9%

CASE QUESTIONS

1. Is she becoming hypoglycemic?
2. How can we confirm that her episodes are as a result of hypoglycemia?
3. What causes these spells?
4. How can the spells be prevented?

ANSWERS AND EXPLANATIONS

1. Hypoglycemia is typically defined in diabetes as a glucose level below 70 mg/dL. The complete definition of hypoglycemia is the triad of (1) signs and symptoms of hypoglycemia; (2) a blood glucose measured to be low; and (3) resolution of those symptoms with treatment.[1] Innate counterregulatory physiologic responses start at a glucose level of 70 mg/dL to protect from further drops in blood sugar. Progressive hypoglycemia below this threshold poses an increased health risk for the person.[2,3]

   People without any glucose or insulin abnormalities can have glucose readings in the 60s mg/dL, particularly at night.[4] This is because physiologic glucose management during fasting and while asleep is a balance between hepatic glucose release and pancreatic insulin production. Typically, the liver generates just enough glucose to meet the basal metabolic needs of the body (primarily the brain) and pancreatic insulin production is just enough to assist in the cellular uptake of available glucose.

   Symptomatic hypoglycemia is defined by Whipple triad: a measured glucose less than 55 mg/dL, typical signs and symptoms of hypoglycemia, and resolution of symptoms with normalization of glucose.[1] Hypoglycemia is relatively uncommon in people who are not taking antidiabetic medications, as the body possesses multiple physiologic layers of defense to prevent hypoglycemia from occurring (Table 5.1). Ironically, the body has fewer defenses to prevent hyperglycemia. Symptomatic hypoglycemia, while very distressing for the patient, is rarely

TABLE 5.1 Physiologic Response to Hypoglycemia[5,6]		
Glucose Level	**Response**	**Result**
80-85 mg/dL	Suppression of insulin secretion	Primary defense—stops most
65-70 mg/dL	Increased glucagon secretion	Primary counterregulatory response
	Increased secretion of epinephrine	Primary response for those who do not take insulin
60 mg/dL	Increase in cortisol and growth hormone	Slower system: minor role
50-55 mg/dL	Hunger	Increase in exogenous glucose
<50 mg/dL	Neuroglycopenic S/S	Compromises further responses

dangerous to someone who does not have diabetes. However, hypoglycemia can be immediately life-threatening.

The patient presenting in this scenario has typical symptoms; however, it is necessary to confirm that she is indeed becoming hypoglycemic and identify a cause if possible.

2. There are many things other than hypoglycemia that could cause this patient's symptoms (dysrhythmias, hypotension, seizures, etc). This patient's fingerstick glucose helps to narrow our differential. Now we need to focus on her diagnosis.

   These can be determined in several ways. Perhaps the simplest option would be to provide the patient with a glucometer and instructions to check glucose levels upon the occurrence of each "spell." Another option is to have the patient use a CGM and maintain a log of when she is symptomatic. There are professional versions of CGM systems available that will allow the patient to continuously record 7 to 14 days of glucose readings that can either be downloaded or accessed remotely. This is particularly useful as it allows the physician to see if symptoms correspond in time with hypoglycemia. Alternatively, the patient could be asked to complete a glucose tolerance test.

   If hypoglycemic episodes are found, the next step is to understand their relationship to eating. One way to further define hypoglycemia is by the time it occurs. Postprandial hypoglycemia is most likely to occur within 4 hours of ingestion of food. Postabsorptive hypoglycemia is hypoglycemia that occurs in the fasting state and is more likely to present while the person is sleeping (Figure 5.1).

   This CGM download appears to show that this person is dropping low most often after eating. The hypoglycemic spells are relatively short-lived.

3. People with prediabetes typically have insulin resistance and hyperinsulinemia. For many, the initial defect of glucose regulation is a blunted first-phase insulin response. The first-phase response is a rapid, short-duration release of insulin in response to an increase in serum glucose concentration. Subsequently, the initial blunted first-phase insulin release is followed by an exaggerated second phase of insulin release. The second-phase insulin response starts concurrently with first-phase response and typically reaches a plateau 2 hours after the initial rise in glucose. When this second phase of insulin release lasts longer than the glucose rise itself, the person is at risk for "reactive hypoglycemia."

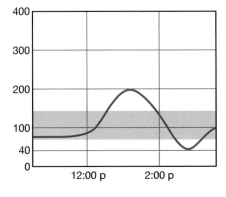

FIGURE 5.1. **CGM for postprandial hypoglycemia.**

4. In general, it is recommended that people with reactive hypoglycemia do the following:
   - Eat 3 to 5 small meals per day
   - Make sure each meal consists of mixed nutrients (carbohydrate/fat/protein) to allow for longer absorption times
   - Avoid simple carbohydrate ingestion alone, as carbohydrate-only meals induce significant insulin spikes leading to rapid glucose uptake followed by second-phase mismatches
   - Avoid intake of alcohol for similar reasons
     While it is antidotal and off label, the use of DPP-4 inhibitors can help reduce the frequency and severity of these spells.
     Finally, if the person has prediabetes, physical activity and weight loss (at least 5%) improve insulin sensitivity and reduce progression to type 2 diabetes and reduce risk of reactive hypoglycemia.[7]

Case Summary and Closing Points

In this case a person with prediabetes was experiencing postprandial hypoglycemia because of a mismatch between glucose absorption and insulin secretion. These types of episodes are often mild, but the symptom severity does not always match the level of the glucose. Assuming that there are no competing etiologies, this patient can be managed with lifestyle changes.

References

1. Whipple's triad. Found in Melmed, S. *Williams Text Book of Endocrinology*. 13th ed. Elsevier; 2016:1582-1607. ISBN 978-0-323-29738-7.
2. International Hypoglycaemia Study Group. Glucose concentrations of less than 3.0 mmol/L (54 mg/dL) should Be reported in clinical trials: a joint position statement of the American diabetes association and the European association for the study of diabetes. *Diabetes Care*. 2017;40(1):155-157. doi:10.2337/dc16-2215
3. Agiostratidou G, Anhalt H, Ball D, et al. Standardizing clinically meaningful outcome measures beyond HbA1c for type 1 diabetes: a consensus report of the American association of clinical endocrinologists, the American association of diabetes educators, the American diabetes association, the endocrine society, JDRF International, the Leona M. and Harry B. Helmsley charitable trust, the pediatric endocrine society, and the T1D exchange. *Diabetes Care*. 2017;40(12):1622-1630. doi:10.2337/dc17-1624
4. Service FJ. Hypoglycemic disorders. *NEJM*. 1995;332(17):1114-1152.
5. Cryer PE. Hypoglycemia-associated autonomic failure in Diabetes. *Am J Physiol Endocrinol Metab*. 2001;281(6):E1115-E1121.
6. Cryer PE, Davis SN, Shamoon H. Hypoglycemia in diabetes. *Diabetes Care*. 2003;26(6):1902-1912. doi:10.2337/diacare.26.6.1902
7. The Diabetes Prevention Program (DPP) Research Group. Reduction in the incidence of type 2 diabetes with lifestyle intervention or metformin. *N Engl J Med*. 2002;346(6):393-403.

Case 2. Defensive Eating

"I have to eat a snack between meals or I get shaky."

A 67-year-old man is being seen for a diabetes recheck. He tells you he thinks things are going well. He has had diabetes for 6 years and has learned what he must do to keep his readings in control. It is very important that he follows a strict daily schedule. For example, if he golfs longer than usual, or if he gets to lunch late, he can get shaky spells. He checks his glucose every morning; it is usually below 100 mg/dL. Recently he has had to increase from eating four to five meals per day to prevent these shaky spells.

Med HX: type 2 diabetes, dyslipidemia (6 years), hypertension (6 years)

Medications: metformin 1000 mg bid, glipizide 10 mg bid, basal insulin degludec 80 units in the evening

Allergies: none

Family Medical History: mother and sister with type 2 diabetes; dad with dyslipidemia and coronary artery disease

Social History: no tobacco, no alcohol, and no recreational drug use; lives with his spouse; likes to golf 3 to 4 times per week.

Physical Exam: Ht. 5′8″, Wt. 194 lb, BMI 29.5, P 84, R 14, BP 132/74

GEN: in no distress

HEENT: normal including thyroid exam

CV: normal

RESP: normal

Diabetes foot exam: pulses +2/2 bilateral, sensation decreased to first and second toes by monofilament, bunions noted to both great metatarsophalangeal joints.

Otherwise: normal exam

Glucose Readings	Fasting
Monday	68
Tuesday	82
Wednesday	158
Thursday	78
Friday	90
Saturday	60
Sunday	72

HbA1c: 5.9%, no evidence of anemia or hemoglobinopathy.

Q CASE QUESTIONS

1. Is he dropping low?
2. What is causing the drops?
3. What are the common signs and symptoms of hypoglycemia?
4. What can be done to prevent hypoglycemia in this patient?

ANSWERS AND EXPLANATIONS

1. A normal fasting blood sugar for someone with diabetes is 80 to 130 mg/dL (4.4-7.2 mmol/L).[1] Based on his fasting fingerstick readings, he is hypoglycemic most mornings. It is important to recognize his symptoms are result of his current medication regimen.

2. This person is taking too much medication and is experiencing hypoglycemic episodes. Both glipizide (sulfonylurea) and degludec (basal insulin) can cause hypoglycemia. In fact, his basal insulin dose is quite high (>0.7 U/kg/d). We could consider him "overbasalized." It is generally ill-advised to utilize sulfonylureas when patients are taking large insulin doses. It is important to note that some of the sulfonylureas are considered Beers list medications and should be avoided in elderly patients.[2] While some of his glucose readings in the morning are ideal, it is highly likely that he is dropping low overnight, which in turn is leading to glucose variability in the morning. He is also experiencing what sounds like hypoglycemia during the day based on his reported "shaky spells."

3. Hypoglycemia signs and symptoms can vary considerably between people and even within the same person. Therefore, it is important to ask patients and their family what signs and symptoms they notice with hypoglycemic episodes. Sometimes the patient's family members will notice changes before the patient experiences symptoms. For this reason, if possible, it is important to obtain information from both the patient and their family (Table 5.2).

   For most people, a combination of adrenergic and cholinergic symptoms will present first. Then, if the glucose continues to drop to the point that the brain does

TABLE 5.2   The Most Common Symptoms of Hypoglycemia[3,4]

- Adrenergic
  - Palpitations (8%-62%)
  - Anxiousness (10%-44%)
  - Tremors (32%-78%)
  - Irritability
- Cholinergic
  - Sweating (47%-84%)
  - Hunger (39%-49%)
  - Paresthesias (10%-39%)
- Neuroglycopenic
  - Confusion (13%-53%)
  - Decreased senses
  - Behavior changes
  - Headache (24%-36%)
  - Lethargy
  - Seizures
  - Coma

not have enough glucose to function, the person will develop neuroglycopenic symptoms. Neuroglycopenia refers to alteration of neuronal function in the brain because of a shortage of available glucose. Many people need assistance once the neuroglycopenic symptoms start.

It is a good practice to ask patients about hypoglycemia at every visit and make sure that they:

1. know how to recognize it
2. know how to treat it
3. have the appropriate supplies
4. This patient needs both a reduction in medication and education about his own safe glucose range. There are a couple of options to reduce his medication. Option one is to start withdrawing the sulfonylurea. This should be accomplished by stopping the nighttime dose first, as nocturnal hypoglycemia can be more dangerous. Then, if needed, we can stop the daytime dose as well. The second option is to reduce his basal insulin. We should reduce his dose at a minimum by 10%. However, considering how high his basal dose is, a 20% reduction is reasonable.

Patients are empowered when they participate in the decision-making process. Work with the patient by asking him which medication change he prefers. The main objectives are to help the patient himself become successful while safely managing his diabetes. This is a great opportunity to let the person know that sometimes it is better to reduce medication to enable flexibility in his schedule rather than forcing him to do "defensive eating" to prevent hypoglycemia.

Case Summary and Closing Points

All patients with type 1 diabetes and many with type 2 diabetes will experience hypoglycemia. It is important that patients know their individual symptoms of hypoglycemia and know how to treat this. Hypoglycemia can be very scary for patients, and they will take preemptive actions including omitting medication, or eating to prevent a low before it happens (defensive eating). While these actions will work for that specific circumstance, they often can undermine the treatment plan leading to weight gain and hyperglycemia. Speaking with your patients about hypoglycemia can help to identify other treatment options like changing medication regimens, which can reduce hypoglycemia and not undermine treatment goals.

References

1. American Diabetes Association. Recommended glucose fasting glucose levels. Accessed December 30, 2022. https://www.diabetes.org/healthy-living/medication-treatments/blood-glucose-testing-and-control/checking-your-blood-sugar
2. American Geriatric Society Beers list. Accessed December 30, 2022. https://www.americangeriatrics.org/media-center/news/older-people-medications-are-common-updated-ags-beers-criteriar-aims-make-sure
3. Hepburn DA. *Hypoglycaemia and Diabetes: Clinical and Physiological Aspects.* Edward Arnold; 1993:93-103.
4. Cryer PE, Davis SN, Shamoon H. Hypoglycemia in diabetes. *Diabetes Care.* 2003;26(6):1902-1912. doi:10.2337/diacare.26.6.1902

Case 3. Somogyi Effect

"Why do my morning glucose readings change?"

A 48-year-old man presented for a diabetes recheck. He was diagnosed with diabetes 4 years ago. At first, he was able to control his diabetes and meet his A1c goals via lifestyle modification and oral medication. He is worried that his medications may now be causing his diabetes to be worse. Since we added more medication his first AM glucose readings have become erratic and have started to climb.

He has tried to closely manage his diet and repeat the same schedule of activities each day to see if this will control his glucose readings but without success. He has no idea why his glucose varies from one morning to the next. The highs are really frustrating him.

He was first diagnosed from screening labs 4 years ago following an annual physical. He went to diabetes education and was started on metformin. Then he had a rough couple of years with his asthma. He required several hospitalizations for intravenous corticosteroid treatment and had several oral courses of steroids as well. During one of his hospitalizations basal insulin was started as well. Several months ago, a glucagon-like peptide-1 receptor agonist (GLP-1RA [dulaglutide]) was added, and last month his dose was increased to 1.5 mg weekly. With the change in medication, his A1c has improved from 7.2% to 6.4%.

Med HX: type 2 diabetes, hypertension, asthma

Medications: metformin XR 2000 mg at night, insulin detemir 50 units at night, dulaglutide 1.5 mg weekly; symbicort 80/4.5 2 puffs BID and PRN

Allergies: none

Family Medical History: strong family history (FH) of type 2 diabetes; dad died from a heart attack

Social History: lives with his spouse; works as a schoolteacher; no tobacco or alcohol; walks with spouse in the evenings

Physical Exam: Ht. 5′4″, Wt. 154 lb, BMI 26.4, P 84, R 14, BP 132/74

GEN: in no distress

HEENT: normal including thyroid exam

CV: normal

RESP: normal

Otherwise: normal exam

Labs: HbA1c 6.4%, otherwise normal

Glucose Logs:

Glucose Readings	Fasting	Bedtime
	68	
Monday	192	88
Tuesday	104	
Wednesday	78	128
Thursday	137	112
Friday	58	151
Saturday	162	140
Sunday	149	

 CASE QUESTIONS

1. Why did his glucose readings get worse in the AM?
2. What can be done to capture the change in glucose?
3. How can we address the fasting glucose variability?

 ANSWERS AND EXPLANATIONS

1. This patient is correct in assuming that his high AM blood sugar readings may be related to the increase in medication. For most people with type 2 diabetes, the morning glucose is relatively stable. First AM readings can increase from late evening calorie consumption, increased stress, or even a poor night of sleep. However, as in this patient, they can occur in response to medication changes. Until recently the patient was using metformin and insulin to manage his diabetes. When the GLP-1RA was added to his regimen, his HbA1c improved, but his fasting glucose levels appeared to have increased. It is very likely that he is having nocturnal hypoglycemia with rebound early am hyperglycemia. This hypoglycemia may not be directly related to the GLP-1RA but the interaction of this medication and insulin if it was not reduced when the GLP-1RA was started. This is known as the Somogyi effect.[1]

   When a person has high glucose variability in the AM, despite a stable daily schedule and medication regimen, a search for nocturnal hypoglycemia and am hyperglycemia should be pursued. A clue this patient is experiencing Somogyi-related hypoglycemia is that his HbA1c of 6.4% equates to an estimated average glucose of about 105 mg/dL. This does not match his fingerstick readings and shows that his average glucose is lower than what his fingerstick log reflects.

   Other situations that can also present with hyperglycemia in the morning include the Dawn phenomenon[1] and persistent hyperglycemia due to inadequate treatment. The Dawn phenomenon differs from the Somogyi effect in that it is not preceded by an episode of hypoglycemia. The Dawn phenomenon occurs when exogenous insulin activity is not able to offset hepatic glucose production. Both conditions are more likely to present with consistent fasting hyperglycemia, and low glucose variability. A CGM is a powerful tool to illustrate both situations.

2. To identify glucose level changes that occur during the night, the patient could check his glucose at bedtime, at 3 AM, and first thing in the morning. Clearly this is inconvenient. Obtaining this information is better achieved by continuous glucose monitoring, which would capture the necessary data. If on the mornings that he has high readings, and his blood sugar is much lower at 3 AM, it is likely that he has hypoglycemic episodes overnight and his body "rescued" him by increasing glucagon, epinephrine, cortisol, and growth hormone release to promote gluconeogenesis and raise his glucose.

   This is a dangerous situation and needs to be addressed. We need to either decrease his basal insulin dose or his GLP-1RA dose. It is important to note which basal insulin a patient is using. Insulin degludec, glargine, and detemir have relatively flat basal activity. However, NPH (neutral protamine Hagedorn) does have a peak activity that varies in timing and may cause early AM hypoglycemia (see Figures 5.2 and 5.3 and Table 5.3).

3. For this patient, he was more concerned about the hyperglycemia than the hypoglycemia. This is an important opportunity to educate about the safety concerns with hypoglycemia.

   Since the main issue in this case is actually hypoglycemia, a reduction in medication is necessary. Based on the history of medication changes, one might infer that the GLP-1RA is the medication causing the hypoglycemia. However, the cause and effect are more complicated. When the GLP-1RA was added, it helped potentiate glucose-dependent pancreatic insulin release and increase insulin sensitivity.[2] This class has a very low risk of hypoglycemia when used alone. However, when these medications are added to medications that are known to have caused hypoglycemia, the risk increases. Obviously, insulin has a strong association with hypoglycemia. However, GLP-1As also lower glucose by decreasing hepatic gluconeogenesis. This is an important detail.

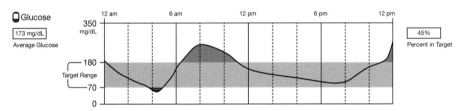

FIGURE 5.2. CGM showing the Somogyi effect.

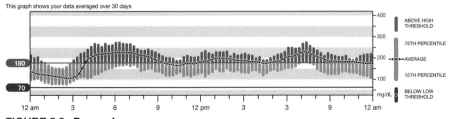

FIGURE 5.3. Dawn phenomenon.

TABLE 5.3	Comparing the Dawn Phenomenon With Somogyi Effect	
Feature	**Dawn Phenomenon**	**Somogyi Effect**
Descriptive feature	Recurring first AM hyperglycemia	Rebound AM hyperglycemia in response to overnight hypoglycemia
Etiology	Reduced insulin secretion 3-5 AM, coupled with increased secretion of insulin-resisting hormones early am	Nocturnal hypoglycemia due to excessive exogenous insulin
Susceptible people	Type 1 and type 2	Type 1 and insulin requiring type 2
Diagnostic evaluation	Measure serial bedtime, 3 AM, and first AM glucose OR use a CGM	Measure serial bedtime, 3 AM, and first AM glucose OR use a CGM
Expected finding	3 AM and first AM glucose high	3 AM glucose low and first AM glucose high and variable
Prevention/ treatment	Increase insulin sensitivity by evening moderate-intensity exercise, increase protein intake in evening, use intermediate insulin or insulin pump	Reduce exogenous insulin

When adding medications to patients already using insulin, the risk of hypoglycemia can be identified by increasing glucose monitoring. In this case we would likely have been able to reduce the dose of insulin while increasing the dose of GLP-1RA. This combination provides excellent glucose control and can reduce some of the unwanted effects of insulin (eg, weight gain). Not uncommonly, it is possible to reduce the basal insulin dose by as much as 30% when a therapeutic dose of a GLP-1RA is achieved. Using insulin and GLP-1RA together can be a powerful method to treat diabetes.

In this patient, a CGM was placed and it documented nocturnal hypoglycemia. The patient was advised to reduce his insulin dose. He was excited to take less insulin but was worried about losing control of his glucose.

The patient's insulin was reduced by 5 units each week until his morning glucose was consistently at goal. He was able to reduce his insulin by 50% to 25 units daily. He maintained the same metformin and dulaglutide doses.

Case Summary and Closing Points

Fasting hyperglycemia and glucose variability can be frustrating for patients and a real challenge for clinicians. It is paramount to figure out what is causing this. If this is related to the Dawn phenomenon, more medication may be necessary, but if it is from the Somogyi effect, the solution is less medication. Utilizing BeAM (bedtime-to-am) glucose readings can really help. Adding a 3-AM glucose or use of continuous glucose monitoring can shed light on this clinical challenge.

References

1. Rybicka M, Krysiak R, Okopień B. The dawn phenomenon and the Somogyi effect—two phenomena of morning hyperglycaemia. *Endokrynol Pol.* 2011;62(3):276-284.
2. Muskiet MHA, Tonneijck L, Smits MM, et al. GLP-1 and the kidney: from physiology to pharmacology and outcomes in diabetes. *Nat Rev Nephrol.* 2017;13(10):605-628. doi:10.1038/nrneph.2017.123

Case 4.   Dawn Phenomenon

"Why do I wake up high even if I do not eat at night?"

A 53-year-old woman presented for a diabetes recheck. She was frustrated because she could not seem to get her fasting glucose down to where she wants it. She was diagnosed with type 2 diabetes mellitus 1 year ago. Her initial am glucose readings were around 200 mg/dL and her HbA1c at diagnosis was 8.9%. She went to diabetes education, made lifestyle changes, and started taking metformin. This seemed to work at first but seems to have stalled.

She takes the maximum dose of metformin she can tolerate. The immediate release gave her an upset stomach and diarrhea. She did better on the extended-release metformin but had problems at doses higher than 1500 mg daily. She even tried splitting her extended-release metformin, taking it twice a day, but this did not help. She was worried she was eating too much at dinner, so she reduced the size of her dinner and even stopped eating after 6 PM, but this too did not seem to help.

For the past 6 months she has not been able to get her fasting glucose below 150 and the rest of the day it is between 130 mg/dL and 180 mg/dL. She has not had any hypoglycemic episodes. She also has not been able to get her A1c below her goal of 7.0%.

Med HX: type 2 diabetes, dyslipidemia

Medications: metformin ER 1500 mg daily, pravastatin 40 mg daily

Allergies: none

Family Medical History: strong FH of type 2 diabetes; mom has chronic obstructive pulmonary disease (COPD)

Social History: lives with her spouse; works as a university professor; no tobacco or alcohol; participates in group exercise classes daily

Physical Exam: Ht. 5′6″, Wt. 167 lb, BMI 27.0, P 84, R 14, BP 132/74

GEN: in no distress

HEENT: normal including thyroid exam

CV: normal

RESP: normal

Otherwise: normal exam

Glucose logs:

A1c: 7.6%

Glucose Readings	Fasting	Bedtime
	138	116
Monday	129	136
Tuesday	118	122
Wednesday	140	134
Thursday	137	112
Friday	125	151
Saturday	142	140
Sunday	149	124

Fasting Labs:

Comprehensive Metabolic Panel	Value	Reference Range
Sodium	138	136-145 mmol/L
Potassium, serum	4.1	3.5-5.3 mmol/L
Chloride, serum	104	98-110 mmol/L
Carbon dioxide (CO_2)	24	19-30 mmol/L
Urea nitrogen, blood (BUN)	21	7-25 mg/dL
Creatinine, serum	0.8	0.5-1.10 mg/dL
eGFR	98	>60 mL/min/1.73 m^2
Glucose, serum	185	65-99 mg/dL
Calcium, serum	9.0	8.6-10.2 mg/dL
Protein, total	7.1	6.1-8.1 g/dL
Albumin	4.3	3.6-4.1 g/dL
Globulin	2.8	1.9-3.7 g/dL
AST (SGOT)	20	10-35 U/L
ALT (SGPT)	22	6-29 U/L
Bilirubin, total	0.7	0.2-1.2 mg/dL
Alkaline phosphatase	100	33-115 U/L

Lipid Panel	Value	Reference Range
Cholesterol, total	194	125-200 mg/dL
Triglycerides	254	<150 mg/dL
LDL (calculated)	100	<130 mg/dL
HDL cholesterol	40	>40 mg/dL men; >50 women
Non-HDL cholesterol	122	<130

Other Labs	Value	Reference Range
HbA1c	7.6%	<5.7% (normal)
Urine albumin/creatinine ratio (UACr)	54 mg/G	<30 mg/G

 ## CASE QUESTIONS

1. What is causing her fasting hyperglycemia?
2. What causes the Dawn phenomenon?
3. What can be done to improve her fasting glucose?

 ## ANSWERS AND EXPLANATIONS

1. Despite being relatively new to diabetes, this patient has done a great job of managing the disease. Her nonfasting glucose goals are largely controlled due to the lifestyle changes she has made. However, her fasting blood sugars are consistently elevated and her A1c is high.

   It is unlikely that she is experiencing rebound morning hyperglycemia. She is only taking metformin, has no known liver or kidney disease, and does not drink alcohol. She has checked her glucose levels at bedtime, at 3 AM, and upon waking, and confirmed that she was not dropping at night, only climbing in the AM. This is the "Dawn phenomenon."[1]

2. The body undergoes several physiologic changes when a person transitions from "day" (awake) to "night" (sleep) and back to "day" (awake). Insulin sensitivity (how sensitive the body is to insulin) is the greatest while we sleep, for most people, typically between 10 PM and 3 AM. In a person without diabetes, this results in the lowest levels of insulin secretion to match the low levels of hepatic glucose production required for basal metabolic activity while sleeping.[1]

   Other hormonal changes occur during the sleep-wake transition. As part of the normal circadian rhythm, cortisol levels dip at bedtime and increase in a pulsatile fashion during the early morning, peaking shortly after awakening. At the same time, growth hormone levels increase as well. Growth hormone increases glucose production through gluconeogenesis and glycogenolysis. These physiologic changes promote insulin resistance. A person without diabetes can compensate for this, as the body increases insulin secretion to overcome this resistance. However, people with type 2 diabetes may experience morning hyperglycemia as they lose the ability to overcome insulin resistance. This is a common source of frustration and confusion for people with diabetes. It is not clear to them why their glucose is high since they have not eaten since the night before. Helping patients understand this can really help reduce this frustration.

3. There are several strategies that could be used to target high fasting glucose levels. Our patient has already tried some actions that often work. Not eating too late at

night is important. If one is choosing to eat at night, it is important to include a protein source to prevent insulin surges. Another option is to engage in moderate intensity aerobic activity. The type and intensity of exercise is important as resistance training and high-intensity physical activity can increase glucose levels.

Often, the reality in patients with Dawn phenomena is they are undermedicated. Medications that can improve fasting glucose include metformin, pioglitazone, basal insulin, sodium-glucose cotransporter-2 (SGLT-2) inhibitors, and GLP-1RA. She has tried metformin but cannot take any dose higher than 1500 mg daily. Pioglitazone is an excellent option to lower fasting glucose as thiazolidinediones (TZDs) focus on improvement of insulin sensitivity.[2] Basal insulin primarily lowers fasting glucose. SGLT-2 inhibitors and GLP-1RA lower both fasting and postprandial glucose.

When choosing between these options, it is important to include the patient in the decision-making process. The patient featured in this scenario decided to start pioglitazone. She liked the idea of addressing the pathophysiology of insulin resistance and the fact that it can lower triglycerides as well. She chose to address the possible increased osteoporosis risk with TZDs by ensuring she had adequate calcium and vitamin D intake.[3] She also liked the idea of taking a 30-minute walk after dinner to help lower her glucose and help maintain her bone strength. This regimen worked well for her. She was able to get her fasting glucose to 110 mg/dL and her HbA1c to 6.3%.

Case Summary and Closing Points

The fasting glucose is often the hardest for patients to get to goal and is often the most frustrating as they do not understand how the glucose climbs overnight even if they are not eating. Informing patients about hepatic glucose production at night is important. Further, letting patients know that normal circadian rhythms of endocrine hormones will cause an increase in insulin resistance first AM, and in people with diabetes this will result in fasting hyperglycemia. Fasting hyperglycemia from the Dawn phenomenon is often one of the hardest glucose to address. Improving insulin resistance or replacing insulin with a peak to match that time of the morning are great ways to address the Dawn phenomenon.

References

1. Rybicka M, Krysiak R, Okopień B. The dawn phenomenon and the Somogyi effect: two phenomena of morning hyperglycaemia. *Endokrynol Pol.* 2011;62(3):276-284.
2. DeFronzo RA, Inzucchi S, Abdul-Ghani M, Nissen SE. Pioglitazone: the forgotten, cost-effective cardioprotective drug for type 2 diabetes. *Diab Vasc Dis Res.* 2019;16(2):133-143. doi:10.1177/1479164118825376
3. Viscoli CM, Inzucchi SE, Young LH, et al; IRIS Trial Investigators. Pioglitazone and risk for bone fracture: safety data from a randomized clinical trial. *J Clin Endocrinol Metab.* 2017;102(3):914-922. doi:10.1210/jc.2016-3237.

Case 5. Hypoglycemic Unawareness

"I don't feel it till I am 40."

A 34-year-old man with type 1 diabetes presented for an exam to renew his driver's license. He had type 1 diabetes for 20 years. His A1c's have typically been well controlled; however, he does have a few lows per week. He is currently taking insulin glargine 36 units each day, and insulin aspart starting at 4 units per meal plus extra if he "feels high." If he drops too low, he skips his insulin at the next meal. He does not check his blood sugar on a consistent basis, because he feels like he can tell how high or low his blood sugar is based on how he feels.

He apologized for being late to today's visit. He ran from work because his car is in the shop being repaired.

He does not have other people who help him with his lows and has not carried glucagon in years. He does keep candy with him to treat mild lows.

Med HX: type 1 diabetes, hypothyroidism

Medications: insulin glargine 36 units daily, insulin lispro about 4 units per meal, levothyroxine 88 μg daily

Allergies: none

Family Medical History: mom—colon cancer, dad—COPD

Social History: lives alone; works in a coffee shop

Physical Exam: Ht. 5′9″, Wt. 127 lb, BMI 18.8, P 84, R 14, BP 132/74

GEN: in no distress

HEENT: normal including thyroid exam

CV: normal

RESP: normal

Otherwise: normal exam

His A1c in the office was 8.9%. His fingerstick glucose upon check in was 62 mg/dL. The medical assistant recommended that he eat 15 g of carbs, but the patient said, "62 is ok—I do not feel low until I am in the 40s." When the physician arrived in the room shortly afterward, the patient was unconscious and beginning to seize. His repeat glucose was 38 mg/dL.

Ⓠ CASE QUESTIONS

1. How common is hypoglycemia in people with type 1 diabetes?
2. Why is he not having any symptoms with his hypoglycemia?
3. How can "hypoglycemic unawareness" be treated?
4. Why was his glucose checked in the office?
5. What is the appropriate acute treatment for this patient?
6. What other actions can help this patient?

ANSWERS AND EXPLANATIONS

1. Hypoglycemia is the rate limiting factor for the treatment of diabetes. It is incredibly common in people with type 1 diabetes with a frequency averaging 2 episodes per week, and 1 severe episode per year.[1] A severe episode is defined as an event in which the person is unable to address their hypoglycemia themselves and need the assistance of others to save their life.

   As mentioned earlier in this chapter, hypoglycemia is usually caused by a diabetes medication, most commonly insulin, a sulfonylurea, or meglitinide. The risk of a patient experiencing a hypoglycemic episode increases 20-fold with insulin treatment and 4- to 5-fold with oral hypoglycemic agents.[2,3] Hypoglycemia is dangerous and potentially life-threatening; hypoglycemia causes 4% to 10% of diabetes deaths.[4,5]

   When treating people with type 1 diabetes, it is important to ask about hypoglycemia at every visit and to make sure the patient is prepared to respond effectively to a hypoglycemic episode.

2. It was mentioned earlier that there are multiple layers of defense to prevent against hypoglycemia. Table 5.1 in Case 1 of this Chapter People with type 1 diabetes lose the first and the second layers of defense. People with type 1 diabetes have lost pancreatic beta cell function; they are not able to produce insulin or regulate insulin secretion. They are dependent on exogenous insulin for glucose regulation. Second, insulin and glucagon have coordinated secretion. With the absence of normal insulin secretion, the coupled control of glucagon is abnormal. This means that the first line of defense against hypoglycemia for a person with type 1 diabetes is the release of epinephrine. Epinephrine is an effective counterregulatory response for hypoglycemia. It increases glycogenolysis and gluconeogenesis at the liver, reduces glucose uptake and utilization and increases glycolysis by muscle, and increases lipolysis in adipose tissue.[6]

   There are several common symptoms associated with activation of the autonomic nervous system because of enhanced epinephrine levels, including tremors, palpitations, sweating, and feeling anxious or irritable. Importantly, the epinephrine response becomes blunted with recurrent episodes of hypoglycemia. This means that each occurrence can lower the glycemic set point before a person's body will release epinephrine and raise glucose levels.

   To complicate matters further, patients with type 1 diabetes may develop a blunted awareness of the epinephrine surge. They may lack the typical signs, symptoms, or cardiovascular reflex abnormalities suggestive of hypoglycemia. When this occurs on a repeated basis the patient may develop hypoglycemia-associated autonomic failure. The patient no longer has enhanced epinephrine response in the face of dropping blood sugars. In the absence of typical symptoms alerting the patient to address hypoglycemia, neuroglycopenic symptoms become the first manifestations of hypoglycemia.[7] These patients have become hypoglycemia unaware (see Table 5.1).

3. When a person has multiple episodes of hypoglycemia and the physiologic epinephrine response is blunted, the person will start dropping low and will not feel

symptoms until they are very hypoglycemic. This is known as "hypoglycemic unawareness." This is one of the most dangerous situations in a person with diabetes. While it can occur in any patient with diabetes, it is much more common in those with type 1 diabetes.[1] It is worth noting that hypoglycemic unawareness increases a person's risk for hypoglycemia 25-fold[1] and is the leading cause of hypoglycemic-associated death in people with diabetes.

Fortunately, hypoglycemic unawareness, once recognized, is treatable. To do so requires a reduction in insulin and permissive hyperglycemia for a minimum of 3 weeks. By stopping all episodes of hypoglycemia, we allow the body to "reset" the threshold for hypoglycemia symptoms.[8] While this may sound counterintuitive to many people with diabetes, this approach can be lifesaving.

4. Any clinical interaction with a patient with diabetes should include a glucose reading. This promotes a discussion of their current state and can be an opportunity to review the signs and symptoms of hypoglycemia. There are anecdotes of patients who go to healthcare visits, are either hypoglycemic during the visit or immediately afterward, and then die in an auto accident. While each patient is responsible for managing their own diabetes, it is recommended that health care professionals be aware of every person's glucose status at the time of care.

5. The treatment of hypoglycemia is based upon the severity of the episode and the location where it happened. For people who suffer hypoglycemia away from a health care setting or in a health care office, the "rule of 15s" should be the first step in self-treatment. This means they should ingest 15 g of a fast-acting glucose and recheck their blood glucose in 15 minutes.

Any patient on insulin should always have a source of carbohydrates with them. This will allow immediate treatment of a hypoglycemic episode. It is useful to provide patients with a list of items that constitute a proper "rule of 15" treatment (see "Sample list of 15 grams of fast-acting carbohydrates"). Many patients incorrectly choose foods like peanut butter crackers or milk as their treatment. While these items may be high in carbohydrates, the protein and fat content in them can delay the absorption of glucose and prolong the hypoglycemia episode.

Sample list of 15 g of fast-acting carbohydrates:
- 1 small piece of fruit
- 1 small box of raisins
- 1 tablespoon of sugar, honey, or corn syrup
- 1 tube instant glucose gel
- 3 peppermint candies (not sugar-free)
- 3 to 4 glucose tablets (check the instructions)
- 4 ounces (half-cup) of juice or regular soda (not diet)

The other part of the "rule of 15s" is that after eating an appropriate 15-g glucose snack the person should wait 15 minutes and then recheck their glucose. This may be hard for many people to do as the epinephrine-mediated autonomic response causes many people to feel a sense of doom, and an urgent desire to eat more. This can result in an overtreatment of hypoglycemia with subsequent hyperglycemia. People can learn how their bodies respond to different foods and may come to self-select a preferred food and carb amount to achieve a reliable response.

If the person has a hypoglycemic episode in which they become neuroglycopenic they will need urgent treatment from someone else. This means those people who are around the person with diabetes on a regular basis should be familiar with the signs and symptoms of hypoglycemia and its treatment. This requires that the person with diabetes share their condition with close family, friends, and coworkers as well as sharing information about when and how they should intervene.

The treatment of choice for severe hypoglycemia in both the community setting and in outpatient health care setting is glucagon. Glucagon administration can be lifesaving. As discussed earlier, glucagon is part of the body's normal defense mechanism for hypoglycemia. When administered as a medication, it rapidly raises glucose levels.

Glucagon, for many years, was only given by the "red kit," a powder that had to be suspended in a liquid and then injected subcutaneously. This was often difficult to administer by a person unfamiliar with injections in nonemergent situations and was very hard to administer correctly during a severe hypoglycemic episode.[9]

There now are multiple easily administered formulations of glucagon. These include a premixed subcutaneous auto-injection, a nasal spray, and a powder that can be constituted into an injectable solution. All patients who have type 1 diabetes (and, in the author's opinion, all people on insulin) should receive a glucagon prescription each year. Most will not be used. The doses that are given will likely save someone's life.

6. For many years, the medical community advocated for very tight control of diabetes to prevent complications. This approach evolved over time, with the recognition that while microvascular complications can be reduced with intensive control, it may come at the cost of hypoglycemia and increased overall mortality. The patient in this scenario would benefit from repeat education on the management of diabetes and best practices with insulin and hypoglycemia. Teaching this patient to achieve a range of glucose control that provides the maximum benefit and minimum risk lets the patient know that lower is not always better.

An important and easily implemented recommendation for patients is to utilize a means to identify that they have diabetes. This includes items such as an ID bracelet, necklace, anklet, or even a tattoo. Some people carry a diabetes ID card in their wallet or purse. This practice of self-identification as having diabetes alerts others that if you are not acting normally or are unconscious, urgently checking glucose and treating hypoglycemia may be needed. Many people are alive today because first responders were able to quickly intervene once it was recognized they had diabetes.

Case Summary and Closing Points

Hypoglycemic unawareness is one of the most dangerous situations that occur in people with diabetes. Clinicians should ask people at every visit if the person with diabetes is experiencing hyperglycemia and what they feel when they drop low. If the person has hypoglycemia unawareness, it is critical that we encourage that the patient stop all episodes to allow the system to "reboot" so the body can respond normally again. These actions can save a person's life.

References

1. Cryer PE. Hypoglycemia-associated autonomic failure in diabetes. *Am J Physiol Endocrinol Metab.* 2001;281(6):E1115-E1121.
2. Amiel SA, Dixon T, Mann R, Jameson K. Hypoglycaemia in type 2 diabetes. *Diabet Med.* 2008;25(3): 245-254. doi:10.1111/j.1464-5491.2007.02341.x
3. Cengiz E, Xing D, Wong JC, et al. Severe hypoglycemia and diabetic ketoacidosis among youth with type 1 diabetes in the T1D exchange clinic registry. *Pediatr Diabetes.* 2013;14(6):447-454.
4. Patterson CC, Dahlquist G, Harjutsalo V, et al. Early mortality in EURODIAB population-based cohorts of type 1 diabetes diagnosed in childhood since 1989. *Diabetologia.* 2007;50(12):2439-2442.
5. Skrivarhaug T, Bangstad HJ, Stene LC, Sandvik L, Hanssen KF, Joner G. Long-term mortality in a nation-wide cohort of childhood-onset type 1 diabetic patients in Norway. *Diabetologia.* 2006;49(2):298-305.
6. Cryer PE. Banting Lecture. Hypoglycemia: the limiting factor in the management of IDDM.. *Diabetes.* 1994;43(11):1378-1389.
7. Tesfaye N, Seaquist ER. Neuroendocrine responses to hypoglycemia. *Ann N Y Acad Sci.* 2010;1212:12-28.
8. Cryer PE. Mechanisms of hypoglycemia-associated autonomic failure in diabetes. *N Engl J Med.* 2013;369(4):362-372.
9. Settles JA, Gerety GF, Spaepen E, Suico JG, Child CJ. Nasal Glucagon delivery is more successful than injectable delivery: a simulated severe hypoglycemia rescue. *Endocr Pract.* 2020;26(4):407-415. doi:10.4158/EP-2019-0502

CHAPTER 6

Anticipating and Responding to Major Life Changes

Introduction

Diabetes is a lifelong condition. And, as with any chronic disease when circumstances change, modifications must be made. This chapter focuses on important transitions in diabetes management that frequently coincide with significant life changes. Being prepared for these transitions can help you and your patients be proactive and thereby avoid some of the pitfalls that might otherwise occur.

Case 1.	Prediabetes and Diabetes Prevention

"I will worry about that when I get diabetes."

A 32-year-old man presents to his primary care provider (PCP) complaining of foot pain. He reports pain in the arches of both feet when standing for long periods of time. It is particularly severe, he reports, when he first gets out of bed in the morning and when he stands after sitting for an extended length of time. The pain improves with walking in sneakers but is worse when he is barefoot. He bought gel insoles, but they have not helped. He has been using over-the-counter (OTC) naproxen for several weeks without improvement in his pain level.

He denies any chronic medical issues. He is not taking any prescribed medications.

Med HX: none

Medications: only OTC naproxen

Allergies: penicillin

Family Medical History: strong family history (FH) of type 2 diabetes; dad and P (paternal) uncle died from chronic kidney disease (CKD)

Social History: lives with his partner. No kids—they have been having trouble conceiving. No tobacco, alcohol, or recreational drugs.

Physical Exam: Ht. 5'9", Wt. 257 lb, BMI 38, P 84, R 14, BP 142/86

GEN: obese man with truncal obesity in no distress

HEENT: normal including thyroid exam

CV: normal

RESP: normal

Extremities: the patient has flat arches and pain with dorsiflexion of toes, pain runs along the plantar fascia of both feet, and has maximal tenderness upon palpation at calcaneus insertion bilaterally

Labs: no recent labs

He was diagnosed with pes planus, plantar fasciitis, and obesity. He was asked to get fasting labs done and advised to check his BP at least 3 times per week.

CASE QUESTIONS

1. What lab tests should be ordered and why?
2. Does he have a diabetes-related diagnosis?
3. What are his other diagnoses?
4. What are the recommended treatments for people with prediabetes?
5. Is there a relationship between his foot pain and diabetes?

 ANSWERS AND EXPLANATIONS

1. This is an obese man with a family history of diabetes and is at high risk for diabetes and should be screened for diabetes. He has a strong family history of renal disease and presents with elevated blood pressure. His renal function will need to be assessed. In addition, he should be screened for nonalcoholic fatty liver disease (NAFLD) as his blood pressure elevation and truncal obesity meet the metabolic syndrome criteria.

   Lab orders should include a CMP (comprehensive metabolic panel) to screen for hyperglycemia, electrolyte abnormalities, renal function abnormalities, and transaminase elevation. A CBC (complete blood count) should also be included since a platelet count is necessary to calculate his FIB-4 score and determine his NAFLD risk. A lipid panel and A1c are important, too, as we suspect he may have metabolic syndrome. Finally, a urinary albumin/creatinine ratio (UACr) would be helpful to identify early kidney disease.

   No specific labs are necessary for his plantar fasciitis. X-rays of his feet could be a consideration to assess for structural deformity and calcaneal spur formation.

   Home blood pressure readings: 152/88, 148/92.

Fasting Lab Results:

Comprehensive Metabolic Panel	Value	Reference Range
Sodium	138	136-145 mmol/L
Potassium	4.1	3.5-5.3 mmol/L
Chloride	104	98-110 mmol/L
Carbon dioxide (CO_2)	24	19-30 mmol/L
Urea nitrogen, blood (BUN)	21	7-25 mg/dL
Creatinine	0.8	0.5-1.10 mg/dL
eGFR (estimated glomerular filtration rate)	118	>60 mL/min/1.73 m²
Glucose	136	65-99 mg/dL
Calcium	9.0	8.6-10.2 mg/dL
Protein, total	7.1	6.1-8.1 g/dL
Albumin	4.3	3.6-4.1 g/dL
Globulin	2.8	1.9-3.7 g/dL

Comprehensive Metabolic Panel	Value	Reference Range
AST (SGOT)	40	10-35 U/L
ALT (SGPT)	42	6-29 U/L
Bilirubin, total	0.7	0.2-1.2 mg/dL
Alkaline phosphatase	100	33-115 U/L

Lipid Panel	Value	Reference Range
Cholesterol, total	194	125-200 mg/dL
Triglycerides	254	<150 mg/dL
LDL (calculated)	100	<130 mg/dL
HDL cholesterol	32	>40 mg/dL men; >50 women
Non-HDL cholesterol	162	<130

CBC	Value	Reference Range
White blood cell count	8.0	3.8-10.8 thousand/μL
Red blood cell count	4.8	3.8-5.10 million/μL
Hemoglobin	14.3	12.6-17 g/dL
Hematocrit	48%	37%-51%
MCV (mean corpuscular volume)	91	80-100 fL
MCH (mean corpuscular hemoglobin)	29.9	27-33pg
MCHC (mean corpuscular hemoglobin concentration)	32.9	32-36 g/dL
RDW (red cell distribution width)	12.7	1%-15%
Platelet count	236	140-400 thousand/μL
HbA1c	6.3%	<5.7%
Urine albumin/creatinine ratio (UACr)	54 mg/G	<30 mg/G
Fib-4 score	0.84	<1.3 (low risk for advanced fibrosis)

2. He has an HbA1c in the prediabetes range and fasting glucose in the prediabetes range. He meets the criteria for prediabetes.

3. His systolic blood pressure, at 142 mm/Hg, meets the criteria for stage 2 hypertension. His serum creatinine and eGFR are normal. Thus, if a UACr repeat check is above 30 mg/G, he will meet the criteria for moderate albuminuria, which would qualify him for stage G1A2 CKD.[1] This could be the result of his prediabetes, his hypertension, or both. Based on his BMI of 38 with other metabolic abnormalities, he should be diagnosed with medically complicated obesity. His elevated ALT suggests a diagnosis of NAFLD, although his FIB-4 score places him in the lower risk category for advancing to nonalcoholic steatohepatitis. As a reminder, one-third of people who develop type 2 diabetes present

with a complication on the day they are diagnosed. Finally, we also diagnosed him with plantar fasciitis at the last visit.

4. There are a wide variety of treatments that have been shown to delay or prevent the diagnosis of type 2 diabetes. Treatment options include intensive lifestyle management, as demonstrated by the Diabetes Prevention Program, several medications, and metabolic surgery.

   The Diabetes Prevention Program has demonstrated a 58% reduction of new-onset type 2 diabetes in those younger than 60 years and 71% in those older than 60 years. The program duration is 1 year and focuses on the achievement of 5% - 7% weight loss via dietary modification and increased physical activity to at least 150 min/wk. It also involves coaching and group classes that can be offered in person or online. Increasingly, these programs are being covered by many insurance plans.

   Medications that help prevent or delay the diagnosis of diabetes include metformin, the alpha-glucosidase inhibitor acarbose, thiazolidinediones, and the GLP-1RAs (glucagon-like peptide-1 receptor agonists).[2-5] To date, no medication has been approved by the FDA (Food and Drug Administration) to treat prediabetes. Historically, metformin has been used most often in people felt to be at high risk for developing type 2 diabetes, especially if the HbA1c is greater than 6.0%.

   In moderately obese persons with prediabetes, bariatric surgery (also known as metabolic surgery) has been shown to reduce the risk of progression to type 2 diabetes to a degree at least twice that of lifestyle interventions. It is worth noting that risk reduction persists for at least 10 years after surgery.[6]

   The patient in this case study has multiple metabolic-related problems. It is important to inform him of the severity of his health risks while also letting him know that much can be done to stop or at least delay their progression.

Intervention	Follow-Up Period	Reduction in Risk of T2D
Antihyperglycemic agents		
Metformin[2]	2.8 years	31% (P < .001)
Acarbose[3]	3.3 years	25% (P = .0015)
Pioglitazone[4]	2.4 years	72% (P < .001)
Liraglutide[5]	3.1 years	66%
Weight loss interventions		
Bariatric surgery[6]	10 years	75% (P < .001) (P value vs placebo)

5. Maybe. Plantar fasciitis often occurs in people who do not have diabetes. However, in people with diabetes who have sustained hyperglycemia, a condition termed "diabetic heiropathy" can arise. Classically, this affects the fingers, though, and is characterized by an inability to fully extend the metacarpophalangeal joints. This

is related to the shortening of tendons and myofascial tissues from glycosylation and can lead to pain, injury, and chronic joint changes.[7]

Case Follow-Up:

The patient was informed that, based on his lab results, he had multiple metabolic abnormalities that were obesity related. In addition, he was told that the presence of protein in his urine suggested he was at risk for progressive kidney disease. The lab results were shared in detail and his options were discussed. He was informed that his relative youth provided him an opportunity to choose any of the above treatments to help delay or prevent his progression to type 2 diabetes. In addition, he was advised that aggressive weight loss would also help address his elevated blood pressure and his liver abnormalities. An emphasis was placed on making proactive changes for "health protection," reinforcing that, at present, his body's systems were working well, and making effective changes now would help sustain his health in the future.

Despite this guidance, he responded that he would "wait and worry about this when and if I get diabetes." He was not motivated to change his diet or increase his activity level. He attributed his elevated blood pressure to drinking too much coffee and subsequently planned to reduce his intake. He did agree to return in 1 month to recheck his blood pressure and repeat his urine albumin level.

Before you react to his response, take the patient's perspective. He came in for foot pain and now he is being told he has multiple medical problems and is likely over-whelmed. It may be worthwhile to try to let him know you will help him to feel better and you want to develop a plan that he can help decide and implement to reduce his risk of these other problems.

Other patients may not be ready to engage. This is a good time to share that you are concerned for their well-being. Let them know that you can be a resource for information and support and when they are ready you will be there to help them. This allows the patient to see you as a partner in health.

Case Summary and Closing Points

Prediabetes affects one-third of all Americans. We know that type 2 diabetes can be largely prevented or delayed. However, doing so requires first that the condition be identified, and second that the affected individual responds proactively. Our role as clinician is to use effective screening strategies, communicate the significance of predi-abetes to our patients, and enroll them in effective evidence-based risk-reduction programs such as the Diabetes Prevention Program or other evidence-based treatments.[8]

References

1. de Boer IH, Khunti K, Sadusky T, et al. Diabetes management in chronic kidney disease: A consensus report by the American Diabetes Association (ADA) and Kidney Disease: Improving Global Outcomes (KDIGO). *Diabetes Care.* 2022;45(12):3075-3090. doi:10.2337/dci22-0027
2. Diabetes Prevention Program Research Group. Reduction in the incidence of type 2 diabetes with lifestyle intervention or metformin. *N Engl J Med.* 2002;346:393-403.
3. STOP-NIDDM Trial Research Group. Acarbose for prevention of type 2 diabetes mellitus: the STOP-NIDDM randomised trial. *Lancet.* 2002;359:2072-2077.
4. Defronzo RA, Tripathy D, Schwenke DC, et al. Pioglitazone for diabetes prevention in impaired glucose tolerance. *N Engl J Med.* 2011;364(12):1104-1115.

5. le Roux CW, Astrup A, Fujioka K, et al. 3 years of liraglutide versus placebo for type 2 diabetes risk reduction and weight management in individuals with prediabetes: a randomised, double-blind trial.. *Lancet.* 2017;389(10077):1399-1409. doi:10.1016/S0140-6736(17)30315-X

6. Carlsson LM, Peltonen M, Ahlin S, et al. Bariatric surgery and prevention of type 2 diabetes in Swedish obese subjects. *N Engl J Med.* 2012;367:695-704.

7. Edrees A. Diabetic cherioarthropathy, a clue for uncontrolled diabetes: case report and review of the literature. *Clin Med Rev Case Rep.* 2020;7:327. doi:10.23937/2378-3656/1410327

8. Prevent T2D Curriculum. https://nationaldppcsc.cdc.gov/s/article/Introducing-the-Revised-PreventT2-Curriculum3

Case 2. Increasing Responsibility in Self-Care

"The diabetes police."

A 30-year-old woman presents for her first diabetes-specific appointment. She is accompanied at today's visit by her sister "Rose." Shortly after introducing yourself, Rose informs you that she does not normally come to her sister's appointments but needed to today because someone had to "tell on her." Until recently the patient lived with their mother, but after their mother's death 6 months ago, the patient moved in with Rose. Rose is concerned that her sister is not taking care of herself. She reports that her sister "eats sugars and does not watch her diet." Apparently, their mother took on the greater responsibility for managing the patient's diabetes. According to Rose, the mother prepared her meals, checked her blood sugars, and made sure that she took her medications. Rose does not have diabetes but has friends that do. They told her that diabetes should be controlled with a "eat nothing white" diet.

The patient, on the other hand, states that she has no problem taking care of herself, and that her sister does not understand diabetes. She does not just eat sugars and tries to pay attention to her diet. She likes to have eggs and toast for breakfast (or oatmeal). Lunch is usually a salad, and dinner is usually soup or salad with meat. She likes to eat rice, but it spikes her sugar too high, so when she eats it, she only eats about half of a cup. She is good about remembering to take her insulin and uses her mealtime insulin regularly. She admits she does not check her blood sugar as often as she should. She gets really frustrated when her glucose climbs for no apparent reason, so sometimes she will just stop checking. She enjoys eating and does not want to be hassled about what she is eating.

She did not bring her glucometer to the appointment, explaining that Rose rushed her out of the door so they would not be late. She promises to bring her meter next time. She feels like her glucose is all over the place, from 50 to 300 mg/dL in the same day. There is no regular pattern that she can identify. She can tell when her blood sugar gets low because she gets shaky and breaks out in a sweat. When she feels low, she drinks juice.

Med HX: type 1 diabetes (14 years), hypothyroidism (10 years)

Medications: insulin glargine 24 units at bedtime, insulin aspart 1:10 carb ratio plus 1:30 above 130 before each meal (often she will estimate the meal and correction)

Allergies: none

Family Medical History: thyroid disorders in mom and sister

Social History: lives with her sister, works in the public library, walks 30 min/d, no tobacco or EtOH.

Physical Exam: Ht. 5'7", Wt. 137 lbs., BMI 21.5, P 84, R 14, BP 118/72

GEN: well adult in no distress

HEENT: normal including thyroid exam

CV: normal

RESP: normal

Extremities: normal pulses, normal sensation to monofilament, and vibration

Skin: no skin changes—injection sites with signs of infection or subcutaneous changes

Point-of-care labs:

Glucose: 248 mg/dL

HbA1c: 7.9%

 CASE QUESTIONS

1. What initial recommendations should be made for this patient?
2. What advice, if any, should be given to the patient's sister?
3. What key information should a person with diabetes share with friends and family?
4. What key information should we review with this patient and her sister?
5. What should be the next steps in treatment?

 ANSWERS AND EXPLANATIONS

1. There is a lot to explore at a patient's first diabetes visit. I often like to open the interview with, "Tell me your diabetes story." This encourages the patient to share information in their own words and not worry about telling the physician what "they want to hear." I encourage the patient to describe how they were diagnosed, what has traditionally worked for them, and what has not worked. Often the patient may also share the positive and negative influences in their life that affects their diabetes management. It is important not to interrupt the patient while they are "story-telling." I follow this up by encouraging them to talk about their activities, interests, hobbies, etc., things they enjoy outside of dealing with their diabetes. Often people with diabetes say they think their diabetes defines them. Patients will be more trusting of caregivers who show an interest in them as individuals rather than diseases.

   I also like to ask what their goals are for the visit. This allows me to prioritize those aspects of care that will best support the patient. I do not always make changes in a treatment regimen on the first visit, especially if I do not have data to support it. My priorities for the first visit are to build rapport with the patient and address their immediate needs. Most patients are more open to treatment changes once they have a sense that their clinician understands their current treatment and is familiar with their past experiences.

From here, I ask the patient about what has worked well in terms of glucose management and at what glucose levels they feel best. (Note that this is not always in the normal range.) Once I have a sense of where they feel best, I explore how often they drop low, what they feel during these lows, as well as how often they go high, and what this feels like. Identifying when and under what circumstances someone is doing their "best" in terms of diabetes management can provide critical information about the support systems that work best for this patient.

I would bring this patient back in a couple of weeks and request that she bring her glucose readings and detailed information about her daily schedule. These will provide critical information from which safe and effective treatment recommendations can be made. Her second visit is also a great time to introduce diabetes technology such as the use of a continuous glucose monitor (CGM) to help us understand her glucose course over the 24-hour period.

One additional factor in this case scenario must be addressed. Part of this patient's "story" is that she has had a diabetes "chaperone" all her life. This is uncommon for someone her age and is likely impacting her ability to manage her condition as effectively as she could. This "chaperone" dynamic is more common in patients with type 1 diabetes, particularly in those patients first diagnosed at a very young age. In this case, it is not clear how or why this pattern of treatment behavior began. It may have been due to resistance among the entire family to adapt to the patient's diabetes diagnosis. It may be related to the patient's own reluctance to assume responsibility for her self-management. Regardless, the dynamic between the patient and her sister indicates that they could both benefit from a visit to a diabetes care and education specialist. The specialist can provide them with a unified set of information to learn from and help them work together more productively.

2. Caring for patients with diabetes and managing their family members' expectations at the same time can be challenging. This may be particularly difficult when the patient is an adult. I want to be able to interact with this patient in a manner that respects her autonomy. At the same time, it is important to acknowledge Rose's concerns, with the understanding that her desire to be present at today's visit is likely motivated by a sincere concern for her sister.

It is important for both sisters to understand that the patient's needs are my priority. As mentioned earlier, this is her diabetes story to tell. In this case, I would ask the patient directly if she is comfortable letting me hear from her sister. This interaction should be brief. I would clearly acknowledge Rose's concerns. At the same time, I would let Rose know that while I appreciate her input my primary focus will be on the patient. Balancing the patient's needs with the family's desires is important; we want everyone's contribution to care to be positive and productive.

Having Rose know that her concerns have been heard and that I will help the patient with diabetes self-management may be a great relief for her. She could have assumed that the patient's health and welfare were her responsibility. Furthermore, asking her to be part of her sister's care team by asking her to participate in diabetes education (assuming this is OK with her sister) engenders trust. Letting her and the patient know I can be a resource for them is crucial.

3. First and foremost, a person with diabetes is in charge of sharing information about their diabetes with friends and family. People with type 1 diabetes make hundreds of decisions every day about their self-care and deciding whom to tell and what to tell is yet one more decision. Supporting personal autonomy and self-disclosure is critical in the patient-provider relationship. People with diabetes who feel that their provider is "autonomy-supportive" show more motivation to regulate their blood glucose levels, which in turn, leads to improvements in A1C levels.[1]

   We recommend that patients share some key aspects with their family and friends.

   1. Know the type of diabetes, its general causes, and general principles of management
   2. How to check their glucose—to help if she is unable to
   3. Know what readings are "too high" or "too low" and she will need help
   4. Know how to identify the signs that she is hypoglycemic
   5. Know and be comfortable treating hypoglycemic emergencies with glucagon and when to alert EMS
   6. What advice and communication styles are most helpful when she is struggling

4. In this particular case, it would be best to start at the beginning with this patient and her sister. This includes clarifying the diagnosis for all involved and making sure that treatment efforts are appropriate for the diabetes type. You want to make sure that the patient and her sister know that this patient has type 1 diabetes and not the other way around, for example. Encourage the patient to speak to her sister about what she needs to help her manage her diabetes. This may feel uncomfortable at first, but voicing her needs and setting boundaries are key to healthy family relationships. Further, emphasizing to the sister that this kind of diabetes is an autoimmune condition and not a dietary-induced condition is needed. That being said, there is much that can be done to help manage the patient's condition.

   The second point of education would be to focus on the baseline entropy that occurs with type 1 diabetes. There are many things that can affect glucose other than food, drinks, and insulin.[2] It is important to let the patient and her sister know that sleep quality, stress, pain, and barometric pressure are just a few items known to affect glucose readings, especially in those with type 1 diabetes.[2] Recognizing this feature allows patients and families to focus on those things that they can control.

   Finally, you will want to work with the patient and family to determine where the lines of responsibility lie. Most adults with type 1 diabetes manage their own diabetes, including glucose monitoring, nutrition, problem-solving, and insulin dosing. Family members often have a secondary role, helping with problem-solving and assisting when severe glucose excursions occur, including hyperglycemia with ketosis and hypoglycemia.[3]

The healthcare team can provide both objective information and resources to help people optimally manage their diabetes. Let them know that there is a whole healthcare team available to help when needed. Other resources include technologies such as smart pens, CGM, and insulin pump systems that can lighten the workload.

Family and friends are often the primary support network for patients with diabetes. There is important information that patients may want to share to help them succeed and help keep them safe. One's diabetes diagnosis is a great place to start. In this case, it is important to make sure the patient and her sister understand that she has type 1 diabetes. Clarifying that this type of diabetes is an autoimmune condition and not a dietary-induced one may help address any shame the patient has about her diabetes, as well as help mitigate the external blame that sometimes family members and friends place on people with diabetes. No one is to blame for their diabetes. The more we can do to address diabetes stigma, starting with our patients and their family members, the better we can support and care for people with this chronic condition.

5. There are a few things that must be done at this appointment:
   1. We need to clarify who is responsible for the patient's insulin injections. Ideally, it should be the patient. Regardless of who is performing the injections we need to confirm they know when to give the injections, how to calculate the patient's dosage correctly, and know how to administer the injections.
   2. It is important that both the patient and her sister are aware of the signs and symptoms of hypoglycemia. This is a great opportunity to review the rules of 15. Most importantly, we want to be sure this patient has a prescription for glucagon and that both sisters understand how and when to use it.
   3. We need to confirm who will have the locus of control and assume primary responsibility for the patient's diabetes care. Once again, it is important for the sister to know you are there to provide guidance and support, but one or both will be managing the patient's diabetes. Because of this family's dynamics these roles need to be clearly established.
   4. The patient's insulin dosing instructions should be reviewed, as should be expectations for self-monitoring. We will want to make sure the patient has prescriptions for everything she needs to administer her insulin and monitor her blood sugar.
   5. We should schedule the appointment for both sisters to meet with a diabetes care and education specialist.
   6. We should briefly discuss the agenda for our next appointment. Our focus at her next visit will be evaluating her glucose control. We will ask the patient to return in 1 to 2 weeks with her meter. Alternatively, if she is open to it, you might place an order for a CGM.
   7. Finally, we want to make sure they both know when and how to ask for help.
   In addition to these items, we will want to make sure the patient has access to her meds, supplies, and refills. We will need more information to know what to do next, so we will ask the patient to return in 1 to 2 weeks with her meter. Alternatively, if she is open to it, you might place a CGM to allow everyone to collect more data from which to build the best possible treatment plan.

Case Summary and Closing Points

Managing one's diabetes can be challenging. Strong social and psychological support can ease the burden of this management. Family and friends can be valuable allies. However, the person with diabetes should have primary responsibility for their care. Taking over someone else's diabetes management is not supporting them. Clearly establishing roles and responsibilities helps promote patient empowerment in diabetes self-management.

References

1. Williams GC, Freedman ZR, Deci EL. Supporting autonomy to motivate patients with diabetes for glucose control. *Diabetes Care*. 1998;21(10):1644-1651.
2. Bright Spots-Factors that affect glucose in type 1 diabetes. Accessed December 30, 2022. https://diatribe.org/poster-now-available-42-factors-affect-blood-glucose
3. ElSayed NA, Aleppo G, Aroda VR, et al; on behalf of the American Diabetes Association. 5. Facilitating Positive Health Behaviors and Well-being to Improve Health Outcomes: Standards of Care in Diabetes—2023. *Diabetes Care*. 1 January 2023;46(Suppl_1):S68-S96. doi:10.2337/dc23-S005

Case 3. Young Adult With Type 1 Diabetes

"Type 1 diabetes 2.0"

A 22-year-old man presents as a new patient to establish diabetes care. He recently graduated from college and moved to the area several months ago to begin a new job. He was diagnosed with type 1 diabetes when he was 12 years old and went into diabetic ketoacidosis (DKA). For the first few years after his diagnosis, he managed his diabetes fairly well. Things went downhill when he started high school. He did not want to have diabetes anymore, so he largely ignored it. He was also diagnosed with celiac disease when he was in 10th grade. Everything he liked to eat made him sick. He was in and out of the hospital several times with DKA. He did a little better while he was in college and was seen periodically at student health. He used what they prescribed for him but did not really monitor his blood sugar or pay much attention to his diet. Now that he has a new job, with health insurance, and a girlfriend, he feels like it is time for him to get better control of his diabetes.

He lost his insurance after graduation and was not able to afford his prescriptions, so he bought some NPH and Regular until he could get in for an appointment. He also bought a meter and has been checking his blood sugars for the past few weeks. He learned to carb count when he was first diagnosed and has been using the ratio they gave him in college. He was not sure what his basal dose should be, so he looked it up on-line and just guessed based on his weight. He has been avoiding gluten and carbs and drinking much less beer than he was in college. He is trying to eat three or four high-protein meals each day, and has been drinking a lot of water. He has been having a lot of highs and some lows. He would like to get on a new treatment plan. He felt pretty good on his prior insulins and wants to know if he can get back on them or maybe even a pump. He is also interested in using a CGM. He brought his meter and log-book with him today so you could see what has been happening.

Med HX: type 1 diabetes (10 years), celiac disease (6 years)

Medications: Currently taking NPH 14 units in the AM and 12 units in the PM and Regular at meals 1:15 carb ratio and 1 per 50 above 200 mg/dL (often will take fixed boluses). Last prescription—insulin degludec 20 units at bedtime, insulin lispro 1:15 carb ratio plus 1:50 above 200 before each meal.

Allergies: none

Family Medical History: none known

Social History: lives with his partner, no tobacco, occasional EtOH, occasional marijuana. No regular exercise, gluten-free diet

Physical Exam: Ht. 5'9″, Wt. 157 lb, BMI 23.3, P 84, R 14, BP 118/72

GEN: well adult in no distress

HEENT: normal including thyroid exam

CV: normal

RESP: normal

Extremities: normal pulses, normal sensation to monofilament and vibration

Skin: no skin changes—injection sites intact without signs of infection on the abdomen, arms, and thighs

Point-of-care labs:

Glucose: 248 mg/dL

HbA1c: 8.8%

Glucose logs:

	Su	Mo	Tu	We	Th	Fr	Sa
Fasting	78	128	85	99	120	105	168
2 hours after B (breakfast)	160	153	188	180			
Before L (lunch)	132	110	95	140	113	103	99
2HPP (2-hour postprandial plasma glucose) L			54			66	
AC D (before dinner)	159	165	140	174	183	155	143
2HPP D (2 hours after dinner)							
HS (bedtime)	130	169	177	156	199	180	174

 CASE QUESTIONS

1. Where do you start with this patient?
2. How do you help him get back to his normal insulin schedule?
3. What other tools can you offer him?

4. What initial screening lab work should you obtain?
5. How do you prevent failure-to-follow-up among young adults with diabetes?

 ANSWERS AND EXPLANATIONS

1. First, congratulate him on his successes and for where he is in terms of building his life. Thank him for sharing his story and establishing care. Let him know your desire is to be a resource to help him achieve his larger health goals. In general, at the first meeting it is important to invite your patients to invest in their own health by forming a partnership with you and your team.

2. The patient has shared with you that he would like to resume his prior insulin regimen. This may be a reasonable starting point; however, we do not know how his control was previously. In general, NPH insulin is dosed 2 to 3 times per day. NPH differs from other basal insulins in that it has a significant peak activity. Depending on when it is dosed it can cover some mealtime glucose excursions. Since we will be using prandial insulin for each meal, we may want to start with a slightly lower basal analogue insulin dose. A reasonable starting point is 80%-100% of the NPH dose. Our patient is taking 26 units per day total of NPH, so we can start him on insulin degludec 22 units dosed once daily.

   There is a 1:1 conversion between Regular human insulin (R) and rapid-acting insulin analogues. We can easily substitute whichever one his insurance covers.

   It is possible that the ratio he learned as a teenager may no longer be correct for him. This is a great opportunity to assess his confidence using a carb ratio and correction scale. If he is comfortable counting carbs, we could ask him if he thinks his ratio is correct. He may have valuable insight regarding his insulin dosage. If he is not sure, we should start with his previous ratio and correction scale, have him closely monitor his glucose readings, and ask him to come back in several weeks to review them together.

   If he is not comfortable with carb counting and using a correction scale, we should encourage him to meet with a diabetes care and education specialist. Revisiting diabetes education could be very useful for him now that he is an adult with new life circumstances. Certainly, his learning needs are much different now than when he was diagnosed. Since he has expressed interest in a pump, it is that much more important that he have specific education and training and be skilled in accurate carb counting.

   In Chapter 2, Case 4,[1-3] there is a list of recommended specific skills I like to share with young adults with type 1 diabetes.

3. He has already expressed an interest in potentially starting a pump and using a CGM. You could introduce him to some of the available options for pumps, smart pens, hybrid closed loop devices, and continuous glucose monitoring systems. If he is interested, send him to the American Diabetes Association website or Diabeteswise.org to review what is available.[2,3] As mentioned previously, these are great subjects to explore more with the diabetes care and education specialist and can be revisited at follow-up.

4. The lab work that we typically order for people with diabetes would include blood tests to assess liver and kidney function, glucose control, lipid levels, and

a urine screen for diabetes-related kidney disease. A blood count can be useful to confirm normal hemoglobin levels for HbA1c accuracy. For patients with type 1 diabetes, it is reasonable to add some additional screening tests for other autoimmune conditions. These include screens for thyroid disease and celiac disease.[4]

This patient has known celiac disease. People with active celiac disease can become deficient in iron, calcium, magnesium, zinc, folate, niacin, riboflavin, vitamin B_{12}, and vitamin D. They may be protein deficient as well. We would want to test these levels too.

People with type 1 diabetes should have the following labs at least annually:
BMP (basic metabolic panel), to monitor renal function
1. Urine for albumin/creatinine ratio (UACr or microalbumin)
2. TSH (thyroid-stimulating hormone), to look for autoimmune disease

People with type 2 diabetes should have the following labs at least annually:
1. CMP, to monitor renal function, transaminase elevations associated with NAFLD
2. Urine for albumin/creatinine ratio (UACr or microalbumin)
3. B_{12}, if on metformin
4. CBC (comprehensive metabolic panel), to assist in assessment for NAFLD and CKD

Periodic labs ordered based on current treatments and control:
1. HbA1c
2. Lipid panel
3. Urine for albumin/creatinine ratio (UACr or microalbumin) (if elevated)

Other screening labs specific to type 1 diabetes:
1. Celiac panel—should be done at least once in a lifestyle—frequency recommendation varies.

5. We mentioned in Chapter 2 that many people diagnosed with diabetes (both type 1 and type 2) as children who received their care via specialty centers have high attrition rates as they transition to adult medical care.[5] To minimize this from occurring, it is recommended as patients age out of pediatric care their specialty team coordinates overlapping care with the primary care or adult diabetes specialty teams. This helps to assure an effective handoff[5] and provides more consistent support for the patient transitioning from dependent to independent self-care regimens.

Unfortunately, the seamless evolution from pediatric to adult management does not occur on a consistent basis. Young adults with type 1 diabetes transitioning out of specialty pediatric care often find their first entry into adult medicine is with a primary care clinician. The first meeting can be challenging for both the patient and the provider. From the patient's perspective the variety of resources they are accustomed to might be lacking. They may notice that no one immediately downloads their data or performs a fingerstick. The provider, on the other hand, may not have a comfort level managing a patient with type 1 diabetes. Most PCPs are comfortable with type 2 diabetes management but are less knowledgeable about complex insulin regimens and the needs of the type 1 patient. My motivation in writing this text is to help bridge that gap.

I encourage you to enthusiastically welcome these patients into adult health care. Encourage them to share their personal experiences and needs. Assure them that PCPs are well-suited to manage chronic disease states, or coordinate care if necessary. Inform them they may need to learn new ways of doing things in the adult healthcare system, but they will not have to do it alone.

Here are a few additional tips to consider that may help make the transition easier for you and the young adult with type 1 diabetes:

1. Put extra time in your schedule for this patient. You will need the extra time to get to know them and review their medical history to make a plan going forward.
2. If possible, work with their pediatric endocrinologist to talk to them and their families about the adult transition. If you are co-located, you can schedule a time to meet in tandem with the pediatric endocrinologist.
3. Arrange peer support meetings with your young adult patients so that they can discuss their experiences together. If you have nurses, social workers, and/or psychologists, invite everyone to meet together to discuss the adult transition.
4. Consider shared medical appointments with your young adults with type 1 diabetes.
5. Be open to contacting young adult patients in different ways. Phone calls and emails may not be the best way to get in touch with them.

Case Summary and Closing Points

Young adults with type 1 diabetes often find themselves meeting with a primary care clinician to help with their diabetes management as their first medical appointment that they do alone. The first meeting can be a startling event for both the patient and the clinician. Primary care is well suited to help provide evidence-based care for people through all their life transitions. This is perhaps most true in the case of treatment for individuals with type 1 diabetes. While many adult-only clinician are not used to pediatric care systems or following people as they mature, family medicine, in particular, do this regularly for their patients.

Encourage your patients to share their personal experiences and needs. Acknowledge at the outset, that you believe they can effectively manage their diabetes. They may need to learn new ways of doing things in the adult healthcare system, but they will not have to do it alone. Diabetes care and education specialists, along with their primary physician, are great resources with extensive experience in training and retraining individuals to maximize the benefits of any treatment plan.

References

1. ADA Support page. Accessed December 30, 2022. https://www.diabetes.org/tools-support
2. ADA Consumer guide. Accessed December 30, 2022. https://consumerguide.diabetes.org/
3. Diabeteswise.org website. Accessed December 30, 2022. https://diabeteswise.org/#/
4. American Diabetes Associations Standards of Care for the person with Diabetes. Chapter 4. Comprehensive Medical Evaluation and Assessment of Comorbidities. Accessed December 30, 2022. https://diabetesjournals.org/care/article/45/Supplement_1/S46/138926/4-Comprehensive-Medical-Evaluation-and-Assessment

5. Peters A, Laffel L, American Diabetes Association Transitions Working Group. Diabetes care for emerging adults: recommendations for transition from pediatric to adult diabetes care systems – a position statement of the American diabetes Association, with representation by the American college of osteopathic family physicians, the American Academy of pediatrics, the American Association of clinical endocrinologists, the American osteopathic Association, the centers for disease control and prevention, children with diabetes, the endocrine Society, the International Society for pediatric and Adolescent diabetes, Juvenile diabetes Research Foundation International, the National diabetes education program, and the pediatric endocrine Society (formerly Lawson Wilkins Pediatric Endocrine Society). *Diabetes Care*. 2011;34(11):2477-2485. doi:10.2337/dc11-1723

Case 4.   Genetics of Diabetes Types

"Should I not have children?"

A 28-year-old woman presents for her diabetes recheck (type 1 diabetes). This has been a tough year for her. At the onset of the COVID-19 pandemic, she began working from home. This provided her with the time to prepare healthy meals and exercise regularly. She took her insulin, checked her blood sugars, and her diabetes control improved. She felt better and was much less stressed.

This all changed in the last year. She had to "re-enter the rat race." She was told to return to the office. She is back to commuting 45 minutes each way. She no longer has the time to prepare healthy meals and is eating on the run again. She is too tired after work to exercise. She is starting to feel overwhelmed and stressed out and knows her blood sugars are high again.

Her life has also become more "complicated." She met someone and is considering a long-term relationship with him but is worried her diabetes will ruin things. She is uncertain how to tell her partner about her diabetes without scaring him or making her look weak. She knows he wants to have a family, but she is not sure if it is safe for her to have children. She also is afraid that if she had children, they would have diabetes too. Right now, they are using condoms. She is afraid to get pregnant and wonders if she should start something for contraception.

She had COVID-19 once about 6 months ago, but it was not very severe. Since the onset of COVID-19 she has gained about 15 lb. Other than that, her health history is unchanged. She has gotten all of her COVID-19 boosters.

She checks her glucose frequently (up to 10 times per day) and pays attention to her readings. She gets alarms when she drops below 70. She has had a few symptomatic lows. She uses her glucose gel when that happens. She always keeps gel or some peppermints with her and has glucagon at her home and work. Her last severe hypoglycemia episode was 1 year ago. She also has glucagon available at home and at work. When her glucose readings go above 250 she gets a headache and feels tired. That has been happening more frequently. She gives herself a little extra fast-acting insulin when that happens.

She considered an insulin pump in the past but did not want something connected to her all the time—"it's like a big shiny diabetes billboard." She is wondering about a sensor as well.

Med HX: type 1 diabetes (14 years), mild background retinopathy

Medications: insulin detemir 32 units each morning, insulin aspart 1:7 carb ratio for breakfast, 1:8 units for lunch and dinner, correction factor 1:25 above 125 mg/dL

Allergies: none

Family Medical History: dad with vitiligo, mom with hypothyroidism

Social History: lives alone with her pet cat, works as a web designer; no tobacco use; drinks wine occasionally; walks at work some days at lunch.

Physical Exam: Ht. 5'6", Wt. 148 lb, BMI 23.8, P 70, R 15, BP 130/72

GEN: in no distress

HEENT: normal including thyroid exam

CV: normal

RESP: normal

Skin: injection sites were largely intact lipohypertrophy noted at injection sites on both deltoid areas

Extremities: normal pulses, good skin care, no loss of sensation to monofilament

Fasting Labs:

Comprehensive Metabolic Panel	Value	Reference Range
Sodium	140	136-145 mmol/L
Potassium, serum	4.2	3.5-5.3 mmol/L
Chloride, serum	104	98-110 mmol/L
Carbon dioxide (CO_2)	24	19-30 mmol/L
Urea nitrogen, blood (BUN)	21	7-25 mg/dL
Creatinine, serum	0.8	0.5-1.10 mg/dL
eGFR	98	>60 mL/min/1.73 m^2
Glucose, serum	112	65-99 mg/dL
Calcium, serum	9.0	8.6-10.2 mg/dL
Protein, total	7.1	6.1-8.1 g/dL
Albumin	4.3	3.6-4.1 g/dL
Globulin	2.8	1.9-3.7 g/dL
AST (SGOT)	30	10-35 U/L
ALT (SGPT)	42	6-29 U/L
Bilirubin, total	0.7	0.2-1.2 mg/dL
Alkaline phosphatase	100	33-115 U/L

Lipid Panel	Value	Reference Range
Cholesterol, total	134	125-200 mg/dL
Triglycerides	58	<150 mg/dL
LDL (calculated)	66	<130 mg/dL
HDL cholesterol	60	>40 mg/dL men; >50 women

Other Labs	Value	Reference Range
HbA1c	6.7%	<5.7% (normal)
Urine albumin/creatinine ratio (UACr)	54 mg/g	<30 mg/g

CASE QUESTIONS

1. What is the risk that her children will get type 1 diabetes?
2. What advice would you give her about possible pregnancy?
3. What are the rates of inheritance for different forms of diabetes?

ANSWERS AND EXPLANATIONS

1. The relative risk of inheritance for type 1 diabetes is actually quite low. A mother with type 1 diabetes has an approximate 4% chance that her offspring will develop type 1 diabetes if she delivers prior to age 25. The risk decreases to 1% if she delivers after age 25. If the father has type 1 diabetes, the risk increases slightly to 4%-7%. If both parents have type 1 diabetes the risk is between 10% and 25%. While this is higher than the risk among the general population at 0.4%, the risk of inheritance is much smaller when compared to other forms of diabetes.[1,2] Sharing this information may alleviate some of her concerns about getting pregnant. Importantly, remember to acknowledge her feelings. Recognizing and acknowledging her feelings can help diffuse her anxiety while also expressing empathy for her.

2. The most important thing she needs to know about having the healthiest possible pregnancy for her and her child is glucose control. The desired HbA1c for women who plan to conceive is <6.5%. Encourage the use of technology, including insulin pumps, CGM, and hybrid closed loop systems. These tools help patients get to glucose goals and often reduce the risk of hypoglycemia as well. These tools will be discussed in more detail in Chapter 7.

    Encourage her to plan the pregnancy. Promote the use of contraception if she and her partner are not ready to have a child.

    We will offer her a professional CGM to try for a 10 to 14 days to see how it feels and how it can help her with her diabetes management.

3. This is a frequently asked question, and a common source of confusion for many patients and family members of patients with diabetes. Therefore, it is important to have this information readily available:

Diabetes Type	Type 1	Type 2	Monogenic Diabetes
Risk for offspring of a person with diabetes	3%-7%	15%-25%	50%

Case Summary and Closing Points

People with diabetes face many challenges that impact their daily life. One large area of concern for many women with diabetes is their ability to conceive and then safely maintain their pregnancy. Encouraging planned pregnancies and establishing A1C targets helps to assure healthy pregnancies for the mother and child. Both men and women of childbearing age often have concerns about passing on diabetes to their children. Helping patients know the potential genetic risk is important and often provides a degree of reassurance.

References

1. Parkkola A, Härkönen T, Ryhänen SJ, Ilonen J, Knip M; Finnish Pediatric Diabetes Register. Extended family history of type 1 diabetes and phenotype and genotype of newly diagnosed children. *Diabetes Care.* 2013;36(2):348-354. doi:10.2337/dc12-0445
2. Turtinen M, Härkönen T, Parkkola A, Ilonen J, Knip M; Finnish Pediatric Diabetes Register. Characteristics of familial type 1 diabetes: effects of the relationship to the affected family member on phenotype and genotype at diagnosis. *Diabetologia.* 2019;62(11):2025-2039. doi:10.1007/s00125-019-4952-8

Case 5. Older Adult

"I am so tired."

A 73-year-old man presents for his annual check-up. Life during COVID-19 has been hard for him.

Two of his close friends died from COVID-19 when the pandemic started. Last year he had a heart attack and needed to have open heart surgery. Recently he was told he has kidney disease. It has been challenging to adjust to the changes in his health and the loss of his friends. Before the pandemic, he was golfing regularly and played cards with his friends several times each week. Now, it feels like he spends more time in hospitals and doctor's offices than he does at home. He does not have the energy to play golf anymore. He spends most of his time alone reading and watching TV. He is frustrated because he feels like his health has declined considerably and seems to be getting worse.

Managing his diabetes has become more of a chore. He has not been checking his glucose as often as he used to. His morning readings are usually in the 150s. He stopped checking in the afternoons and at night because his readings were high. Since he had his heart attack, he is not as active as he used to be. He sits around his apartment and snacks all day and has gained about 15 lb. He knows this is probably why his blood sugars are higher than they used to be.

Med HX: type 2 diabetes, hypertension, dyslipidemia, CAD (coronary artery disease) s/p CABG (coronary artery bypass graft surgery), HFrEF (heart failure with reduced ejection fraction; EF36%), CKD 3a, prostate cancer s/p brachytherapy

Medications: carvedilol 6.25 mg bid, atorvastatin 40 mg daily, Entresto 97/103 mg bid, empagliflozin 25 mg daily, ASA (acetylsalicylic acid) 325 mg daily, insulin glargine 10 units daily, Lasix 40 mg daily am

Allergies: none

Family Medical History: no-contributory

Social History: lives with his spouse; has 2 children and 6 grandchildren; retired civil engineer; no regular exercise

Physical Exam: Ht. 5′5″, Wt. 198 lb, BMI 32.9, P 87, R 19, BP 130/78

GEN: appears older than stated age, obese, in no distress

HEENT: normal including thyroid exam, no jugular vein distention

CV: heart regular, widened point of maximal impulse (PMI) noted

RESP: bibasilar crackles

Extremities: peripheral pulses normal lower extremities, +2 pitting edema bilaterally, mild callusing noted to both great toes, sensation intact to monofilament

Fasting Labs:

Comprehensive Metabolic Panel	Value	Reference Range
Sodium	136	136-145 mmol/L
Potassium, serum	3.8	3.5-5.3 mmol/L
Chloride, serum	98	98-110 mmol/L
Carbon dioxide (CO_2)	28	19-30 mmol/L
Urea nitrogen, blood (BUN)	48	7-25 mg/dL
Creatinine, serum	2.1	0.5-1.10 mg/dL
eGFR	48	>60 mL/min/1.73m^2
Glucose, serum	155	65-99 mg/dL
Calcium, serum	8.8	8.6-10.2 mg/dL
Protein, total	6.1	6.1-8.1 g/dL
Albumin	3.8	3.6-4.1 g/dL
Globulin	2.8	1.9-3.7 g/dL
AST (SGOT)	30	10-35 U/L
ALT (SGPT)	42	6-29 U/L
Bilirubin, total	0.7	0.2-1.2 mg/dL
Alkaline phosphatase	90	33-115 U/L

Lipid Panel	Value	Reference Range
Cholesterol, total	148	125-200 mg/dL
Triglycerides	156	<150 mg/dL
LDL (calculated)	72	<130 mg/dL
HDL cholesterol	44	>40 mg/dL men; >50 women

Other Labs	Value	Reference Range
HbA1c	7.6%	<5.7% (normal)
UACr	288	<30

 CASE QUESTIONS

1. What is your HbA1c goal for this patient?
2. What do you suggest for his diabetes pharmacotherapy?
3. What is his chronic kidney stage?
4. What can you do to help this patient?

 ANSWERS AND EXPLANATIONS

1. Deciding upon one's A1c goal should be a collaborative process between the patient and their provider. Factors impacting this determination should include the patient's age, comorbid conditions, and state of health. As discussed in Chapter 3, the American Diabetes Association's Standards of Care supports looser goals for older patients and those in poor health or with a decreased life expectancy.[1]

    As per ADA recommendation, taking into consideration this patient's age and multiple comorbidities, a reasonable A1c target would be 8.0%.[1]

2. This is an interesting subject to discuss with the patient. Diabetes management has progressed to the point that both glycemic control and extraglycemic benefit need to be considered when selecting medications. When considering this patient's other medical problems (CAD, CKD3, HFrEF), there are several approaches to his diabetes regimen that all have merit.

    1. The first option is to continue what he is currently using, empagliflozin, an sodium-glucose cotransporter 2 inhibitor (SGLT-2i), and basal insulin. His A1c at 7.6% is within his target range. Empagliflozin has good evidence for reducing both his cardiovascular and renal risk. In addition, empagliflozin has FDA approval for reducing cardiovascular death or hospitalization among patients with HFrEF (as well as heart failure with preserved ejection fraction with or without diabetes).
    2. The second option is to discontinue basal insulin and use just empagliflozin. We have already established that he is at his A1c goal. Stopping insulin would likely not change his A1c considerably. This would reduce his medication burden and reduce the expense of his medications.
    3. The third option is to replace his basal insulin with a GLP1-RA. While the basal insulin is certainly helping to control his blood sugar, it does not have

any extraglycemic benefit. The GLP1-RAs dulaglutide, liraglutide, and sema-glutide all have evidence for cardiovascular risk reduction. Since he has established CAD, this is particularly relevant.

One of the key differences between SGLT-2i's and GLP1a's is that GLP1a's are safe and effective in patients with progressive renal disease. Right now, this patient's renal function does not prevent him from being treated with an SGLT-2i. However, if his eGFR dropped below 45 mL/min SGLT-2i would no longer have significant glucose-lowering effect. It could be maintained for its heart failure benefit until an eGFR of 20 mL/min. Considering this, it might make sense to introduce a GLP1-RA now.

3. The recommendations for CKD have recently been updated. The KDIGO initiative uses a heat map to help provide CKD staging. It reflects both the importance of the change in eGFR and the amount of albuminuria to determine the stage and person's risk from diabetic kidney disease.

Our patient has an eGFR of 48 mL/min and a UACr of 288 mg/G so he would have stage G3aA2 CKD (Figure 6.1).

4. This patient has experienced a dramatic change in his life over the past couple of years. He has lost some of his close friends and contemporaries, undergone multiple major medical setbacks, and lost some of the normal daily activities he once enjoyed. He has many reasons for feeling down. Many older adults are already at risk for depression, but this patient's risk is even higher due to the issues mentioned above. Screening him for depression and treating it if present may make a real quality-of-life

				Persistent albuminuria categories Description and range		
				A1	**A2**	**A3**
				Normal to mildly increased	Moderately increased	Severely increased
				<30 mg/g <3 mg/mmol	30–300 mg/g 3–30 mg/mmol	>300 mg/g >30 mg/mmol
GFR categories (ml/min/ 1.73 m²) Description and range	**G1**	Normal or high	≥90		Monitor	Refer*
	G2	Mildly decreased	60–89		Monitor	Refer*
	G3a	Mildly to moderately decreased	45–59	Monitor	Monitor	Refer*
	G3b	Moderately to severely decreased	30–44	Monitor	Monitor	Refer*
	G4	Severely decreased	15–29	Refer*	Refer*	Refer
	G5	Kidney failure	<15	Refer	Refer	Refer

FIGURE 6.1. The KDIGO heat map for chronic kidney disease.[2] (Used with permission from Kidney Disease Improving Global Outcomes (KDIGO)).

TABLE 6.1 Depression Screening Tools for Older Adults				
Screening Tool	**Items**	**Rating**	**Time to Complete (minutes)**	**Cost**
Geriatric Depression Scale (GDS)[3,4]	30	Self-administered	10-15	None
Geriatric Depression Scale 15 (GDS-15)[5]	15	Self-administered	5-10	None
Depressive Symptom Assessment for Older Adults (DSA)[6]	27	Clinician interviewer	10-30	None
Detection of Depression in the Elderly Scale (DDES)[7]	25	Self-administered	10-15	None

difference for him. Given his age, consider screening with a geriatric depression scale. These scales were designed specifically for older populations to measure emotional and behavioral symptoms of depression while excluding symptoms that overlap with dementia or somatic disease (see Table 6.1 for validated scales).

Case Summary and Closing Points

Diabetes management should be individualized. When selecting treatment regimens, we should consider the current health and life expectancy of our patients. While we have strong evidence that effective management of diabetes can reduce both microvascular and macrovascular complications, this often takes time. Patients with limited life expectancy and serious comorbidities may do better with less aggressive treatments. However, there is compelling evidence enabling us to tailor diabetes regimens for patients with cardiovascular and renal disease that may help reduce their risk of progressive disease. This approach is part of providing the right amount of treatment to the right person at the right time.

References

1. American diabetes association. Standards of Care in people with Diabetes. Chapter 13-Older Adults. 2022. https://diabetesjournals.org/care/article/45/Supplement_1/S195/138920/13-Older-Adults-Standards-of-Medical-Care-in?searchresult=1
2. de Boer IH, Khunti K, Sadusky T, et al. Diabetes management in chronic kidney disease: A consensus report by the American Diabetes Association (ADA) and Kidney Disease: Improving Global Outcomes (KDIGO). *Diabetes Care.* 2022;45(12):3075-3090. doi:10.2337/dci22-0027.
3. Yesavage JA, Brink TL, Rose TL, et al. Development and validation of a geriatric depression screening scale: a preliminary report. *J Psychiatr Res.* 1982;17(1):37-49. (GDS).
4. Yesavage JA. Geriatric depression scale. *Psychopharmacol Bull.* 1988;24(4):709-711.
5. Almeida OP, Almeida SA. Short versions of the geriatric depression scale: a study of their validity for the diagnosis of a major depressive episode according to ICD-10 and DSM-IV. *Int J Geriatr Psychiatr.* 1999;14(10):858-865. (GDS-15).
6. Onega LL. Content validation of the depressive symptom assessment for older adults. *Issues Ment Health Nurs.* 2008;29(8):873-894. Depressive Symptom Assessment for Older Adults (DSA).
7. Lopez-Torres-Hidalgo JD, Galdon-Blesa MP, Fernandez-Olano C, et al. Design and validation of a questionnaire for the detection of major depression in elderly patients. *Gac Sanit.* 2005;19(2):103-112. (Detection of Depression in the Elderly Scale (DDES)).

CHAPTER 7

Technology in Diabetes

Introduction

The past few decades have seen an unprecedented advance in technology available for the management and treatment of diabetes. Novel devices have made living with diabetes both easier and safer. It is important for the health care professional to have a good working knowledge of these resources to effectively meet patient needs. Being able to provide individualized recommendations can make a significant difference in a patient's experience living with diabetes. This chapter focuses on the current tools that can improve both patient and clinician experience in diabetes care.

Case 1.	How to Make Your Diabetes Office Visits More Efficient

"How can I possibly do all of these things?"

A 68-year-old woman comes in to discuss her diabetes. She has had type 2 diabetes for about 20 years. She was supposed to have fasting labs done before this visit. She does not drive and must take the bus to get to the office for her blood work. She tried coming for her previsit lab work twice before, but each time she experienced symptoms that prevented her from making the journey. She had to eat to feel better, and since she knew the labs were supposed to be fasting, she just stayed home.

Managing her diabetes has been hard. She thought she had a system that worked for her but lately, she feels as though she never knows what her glucose will do on any given day. She tries to be carbohydrate consistent and might take more insulin if she is going to eat more.

Med HX: type 2 diabetes, hypertension, dyslipidemia, knee and hip osteoarthritis, chronic kidney disease (CKD), nonproliferative diabetic retinopathy, peripheral sensory diabetic neuropathy

Medications: metformin 1000 mg bid, insulin glargine 48 units per day, insulin glulisine 12 units with breakfast, and 10 units with lunch and dinner unless she is sure of the carb content of the meal and then she uses a 1:5 carb ratio. She also takes glulisine for correction with 2 units for every 50 mg/dL above 200 mg/dL, atorvastatin 80 mg daily, valsartan/HCT 160/25 mg daily, gabapentin 300 mg po tid.

Allergies: none

Family Medical History: type 2 diabetes in mom and sister, dad—coronary artery disease, brother—heart failure

Social History: lives with her spouse; retired; likes to do things with her social club

Physical Exam: Ht. 5'7", Wt. 187 lb, BMI 29.3, P 66, R 17, BP 132/68

GEN: overweight female with truncal obesity, in no distress

HEENT: normal including thyroid exam

CV: normal

RESP: normal

Extremities: normal peripheral pulses, normal sensation to monofilament exam, bunions noted to both first toes, callus formation on the ball of the foot

Glucose logs:

109	140	168
128	130	305
167	198	178
151	179	390
328	355	165
123	156	305
158	188	181
160	208	336
196	160	218
145	136	157
134	200	249
120	131	195
195	145	187
163	194	174
161	309	244
136	69	99
110	156	264
144	198	218

Labs: *from 18 months ago*

Comprehensive Metabolic Panel	Value	Reference Range
Sodium	141	136-145 mmol/L
Potassium, serum	4.2	3.5-5.3 mmol/L
Chloride, serum	99	98-110 mmol/L
Carbon dioxide (CO_2)	28	19-30 mmol/L
Urea nitrogen, blood (BUN)	12	7-25 mg/dL
Creatinine, serum	2.6	0.5-1.10 mg/dL
eGFR (estimated glomerular filtration rate)	48.2	>60 mL/min/1.73 m^2
Glucose, serum	168	65-99 mg/dL
Calcium, serum	9.9	8.6-10.2 mg/dL
Protein, total	7.1	6.1-8.1 g/dL
Albumin	4.3	3.6-4.1 g/dL

Comprehensive Metabolic Panel	Value	Reference Range
Globulin	2.8	1.9-3.7 g/dL
AST (SGOT)	40	10-35 U/L
ALT (SGPT)	44	6-29 U/L
Bilirubin, total	0.7	0.2-1.2 mg/dL
Alkaline phosphatase	100	33-115 U/L

Lipid Panel	Value	Reference Range
Cholesterol, total	202	125-200 mg/dL
Triglycerides	186	<150 mg/dL
LDL (calculated)	138	<130 mg/dL
HDL cholesterol	36	>40 mg/dL men; >50 women
Non-HDL cholesterol	165	<130

Other Labs	Value	Reference Range
HbA1c	8.8%	<5.7%
Urine albumin/creatinine ratio (UACr)	376 mg/G	<30 mg/G

 CASE QUESTIONS

1. How do you interpret the glucose logs?
2. How can patient glucose data be assessed more efficiently?
3. What other practices can make visits more efficient?
4. What tools are available to help patients and clinicians assess basal and bolus insulin regimens?

 ANSWERS AND EXPLANATIONS

1. The patient is putting in a lot of work to monitor her diabetes. It is important to let her know that you recognize her efforts. Affirm her for the effort she is making to manage her diabetes and record her blood sugars. Despite this work, several questions still remain.

   What is the timing of her fingersticks? Specifically, are these readings taken before or after her meals? Her log indicates she is having some lows. We need to understand at what glucose level she feels the need to respond, and how she chooses to do so. This might be an opportunity to review the rules of 15s (Chapter 5). She is also having significant hyperglycemia. How is she managing these? Once we understand the landscape in terms of glucose checks and actions, we can go into more depth regarding her awareness of possible trends.

Many clinicians like to have logs available prior to entering the exam room. It can take approximately 5 to 7 minutes to review glucose logs and to determine patterns, trends, and mean values throughout the day. This is a necessary step for insulin management but requires time that, unfortunately, many clinicians do not have. The following sections address additional strategies to help make a diabetes visit more efficient.

It is great that this patient is checking her glucose regularly. These readings are necessary for her to be able to determine her dose of insulin at each meal. The logs as presented to us may be a bit less useful. Given that she is checking her glucose before taking mealtime insulin, we might assume that these readings are before breakfast, before lunch, and before dinner.

Specifically for this patient, I would recognize all of the work she is doing to manage her diabetes and document this to help us to help her. Her morning readings are relatively stable reflecting the basal insulin and her nighttime schedule, but the daytime readings vary widely. We will need to learn more about that.

2. Many patients bring a glucose meter to the office visit for review and the clinician scrolls through readings with the patient. This is time consuming and not an effective way to establish trends. Fortunately, the great majority of glucose meters have the capacity to interface with computers, so data can be downloaded, and individualized reports can be generated. Previously, each product line required proprietary software to do so. There are now universal platforms such as Glooko[1] and Tidepool[2] that help clinicians retrieve data from devices. To use these, the provider or a staff member creates accounts with either Glooko or Tidepool and downloads the software to a computer. Meters that have downloadable capacity come with a cable to plug directly into a computer. You will have to remind your patients to bring this to their visits. I recommend setting up a download station in your clinic and assigning a staff member to oversee the process (see more below). This saves time and lets the clinician view glucose data more efficiently.

While it is not addressed in this case—this is a great scenario to consider using a continuous glucose monitor (CGM; either professional or personal version) to get 10 to 14 days of data to see her 24-hour glucose profile. We will discuss more about CGM in the upcoming cases in this chapter.

Here is an example of a downloaded glucometer report. The report reveals specific information indicating when glucose is being measured, making it easier to identify trends. This is a powerful tool to help tailor patients' treatment regimens.

Home Blood Glucose Log.

	Before Breakfast	2 h After Breakfast	Before Lunch	Before Dinner	Bedtime
Mon		81	127	234	92
Tues	128	203	78	281	167
Wed	123			170	375
Thurs	93				
Fri	45		153	177	253

	Before Breakfast	2 h After Breakfast	Before Lunch	Before Dinner	Bedtime
Sat		135			95
Sun	87			107	123
Mon	58	163	200	83	132
Tues	113	160	136	335	102
Wed		156		143	
Thurs	118				104
Fri	74	115	158	202	315
Sat	267	160	163	210	180
Sun		156		124	

3. Helping people manage their diabetes can be time- and labor-intensive. Below are strategies to help make our visits more efficient:
    1. Create and use an office download station
    2. Utilize a point-of-care HbA1c machine
    3. Utilize a written instruction sheet template
    4. Avoid the need for fasting lab work
    5. Have dedicated diabetes-only visits

Create and Use an Office Download Station

As mentioned earlier, the use of a glucose meter (or CGM) download station can save 5 to 7 minutes per patient visit. Downloaded reports allow clinicians to quickly analyze glucose readings and, thus, more efficiently develop a coordinated patient plan.

Here are a few suggestions to optimize the process:

- Identify a specific staff person to be the "device manager." This person will make sure patients bring their devices to visits and oversee data capture.
- Consider creating a download station in the waiting room for patients to utilize themselves.
- Implement data downloads as part of the check-in process.
- Some devices (like CGMs) will upload to the web. A staff member or the provider can review the data online and generate a report prior to or at the time of the visit. In my own practice, a designated MA (medical assistant) downloads reports from the web on the morning of patient appointments.

Utilize a Point-of-Care HbA1c Machine

For many patients, coming for blood draws in advance of office visits often proves challenging.

Despite established protocols for previsit planning, many patients come to visits without having completed labs. As a result, the visit agenda must be postponed until blood work is completed. This either leads to extra work for clinician and staff to communicate results and discuss regimen changes or a delay in addressing results until the next scheduled appointment.

Having point-of-care (POC) testing within the office considerably improves the efficiency of patient visits. Available options include POC HbA1c, POC UACr, and POC lipid assays. Most devices are CLIA waived, which simplifies implementation. The machines are small and easy for staff to use. Some companies/services will provide these devices at no cost with an agreement for the ongoing purchase of test cartridges. Having access to the results at the time of care provides a "teachable moment" with the patient and allows for timely recommendations and interventions. Most practices bill directly for testing and the service is reimbursable, which can maximize profitability.

Primary care research has supported the use of HbA1c machines in practice. One study completed in the primary care setting found that a POC HbA1c machine reduced therapeutic inertia.[3] Another Canadian Health System study found that the use of POC machines were cost-effective.[4] Another primary care–based study found that POC HbA1c was associated with increased frequency of care intensification and improved patient HbA1c.[5] Patients who received POC testing reported greater patient satisfaction and an enhanced relationship with their health care professional.[6]

Utilize a Written Instruction Sheet Template

I find that much of the advice and guidance I provide is repeated from patient to patient throughout the course of the day. I also know that I am often presenting a great deal of instruction and/or education, which can overwhelm patients and family members. Providing patients with written instructions improves both retention and adherence. In my own practice, we provide written templates that have worked well.

Attached is a copy of our office instruction template. The first page identifies glucose, blood pressure, lipid, and antiplatelet goals, and provides insulin dosing instructions. The second page reviews common diabetes medication classes and titration schedules. The third page serves as a reminder of the quality-of-care metrics needed for excellent diabetes management. The fourth page provides rationales for specific medication selections.

Typically, we provide patients with the first two pages to reinforce dosing and self-monitoring instructions. We use page 3 to help inform patients about best-practice guidelines for comprehensive diabetes care. This helps assure that patients are aware of the recommended preventive services and understand the processes of care. This template was designed specifically for our practice; it may not translate well to yours. Using the template has helped alleviate my workload and patients do seem to appreciate having a bigger picture of their diabetes care.

Diabetes Management

Today's Visit Date

How Often Should I Check My Blood Sugar? _____Times per day
__X__ First thing in the <u>morning</u> before you eat or drink and at bedtime
_____ <u>Before</u> lunch or dinner
__X__ Whenever you feel that your blood sugar is low (experiencing symptoms)
__X__ Always check before injecting a dose of insulin
My basal insulin is _____. My dose is _____units at _____time.

My mealtime and correction scale insulin is _____. I take _____ units for my food _____ minutes or right BEFORE breakfast, lunch, dinner (*circle time and meals*).	
My correction scale is:	____ units if less than 150
	____ units if glucose 151-200
	____ units if glucose 201-250
	____ units if glucose 251-300
	____ units if glucose 301-350
	____ units if glucose greater than 351
I also take:_____ ____.	

Blood Sugar Goals	
A1C Average blood sugar over 3 months	Less than 6.5% 7% 7.5% 8%
Blood sugar <u>before</u> eating	80-130 mg/dL or _____mg/dL
Blood sugar 2 hours <u>after</u> a meal	Less than 180 mg/dL or _____mg/dL

Other Treatment Goals	
Blood pressure	Less than 130/80 mm Hg or 140/90 mm Hg
Aspirin (75-162 mg/d)	<u>Secondary prevention</u>: diabetes and history of ASCVD <u>Primary prevention</u>: may consider if have diabetes, increased CV risk and low bleed risk, ages 40-59 but not recommended for 60 years or older
Statin (based on age and risk of heart attack and stroke in the next 10 years and LDL level)	High intensity Moderate intensity None

Starting Diabetes Medications

Class	Agent	Instructions
GLP-1 Receptor Agonists	Victoza (liraglutide)	Week 1: 0.6 mg daily Week 2: 1.2 mg daily Week 3 and thereafter: 1.8 mg daily
	Trulicity (dulaglutide)	Weeks 1 and 2: 0.75 mg weekly Week 3 and thereafter: 1.5 mg weekly *Can increase to 3.0 and 4.5 mg if needed*
	Ozempic (semaglutide)	Weeks 1-4: 0.25 mg weekly
	Rybelsus (oral semaglutide)	Weeks 5-8 (or longer): 0.5 mg weekly *Can increase to 1 or 2 mg weekly if needed* 3 mg daily on empty stomach and 4 oz of water for 30 days, then 7 mg daily *Can increase to 14 mg daily if needed (after 30 days of 7 mg)*
	Bydureon (exenatide—weekly)	2 mg once weekly at any time of day
	Byetta (exenatide—twice daily)	5 mcg twice daily before meals within 60 minutes *Can increase to 10 µg twice daily after 1 month of 5 µg*
Dual GLP/GIP Receptor Agonists	Mounjaro (tirzepatide)	2.5 mg weekly *Can increase 2.5 mg/wk every 4 weeks if needed*
SGLT-2 Inhibitors	Jardiance (empagliflozin)	Once daily
	Invokana (canagliflozin)	*Pay attention to UTI symptoms and keep yourself hydrated
	Farxiga (dapagliflozin)	
	Steglatro (ertugliflozin)	
DPP-4 Inhibitors	Nesina (alogliptin)	Once daily
	Onglyza (saxagliptin)	
	Tradjenta (linagliptin)	
	Januvia (sitagliptin)	

Class	Agent	Instructions
Insulin	Insulin N (NPH)	Basal/background insulin _____ units
	Toujeo (glargine)	Can be taken at bedtime <u>OR</u> in the morning
	Tresiba (degludec)	
	Basaglar (glargine)	
	Lantus (glargine)	
	Semglee (glargine-yfgn)	
	Levemir (detemir)	
	Insulin R (Regular)	Bolus/mealtime insulin ____ units
	Novolog (aspart)	Inject 15 or 30 minutes before a meal (one to three times daily)
	Humalog (lispro)	
	Apidra (glulisine)	
	Fiasp (aspart)	Bolus/mealtime insulin ____ units
	Lyumjev (lispro-aabc)	Inject right before <u>OR</u> within 20 minutes of a meal (one to three times daily)
Fixed Ratio Injections	Soliqua (glargine + lixisenatide)	Start 16 units daily
	Xultophy (degludec + liraglutide)	Start 15 units daily

Diabetes Process-of-Care Check-Off Sheet (American Diabetes Association)

Screenings			
Annual "Comprehensive" Foot Exam	**Yes**	**No**	**Date:**
Feet should be assessed at each diabetes care visit			
Annual Eye exam	**Yes**	**No**	**Date:**
Subsequent examinations for type 1 and type 2 patients with diabetes should be repeated annually by an ophthalmologist or optometrist.			
Annual Lipid Screening	**Yes**	**No**	**Date:**
Annual Liver (LFT) Screening	**Yes**	**No**	**Date:**
NASH Screening (Fib-4 score)	**Yes**	**No**	**Date:**
Every 3 years or if present with symptoms			

Screenings			
Annual Test for Kidney Function	Yes	No	Date:
Urine albumin (UACr) and eGFR in patients with diabetes and/or comorbid hypertension at diagnosis			
How often should I get my A1C checked?	6 mo	3 mo	Date:
A1C within set goal or <7%, then check every 6 mo			
A1C not at goal or ≥ 7%, then check every 3 mo			
Routine Blood Pressure Readings	Yes	No	Date:
Blood pressure should be measured at every routine diabetes visit.			

Medications		
Should I be on aspirin therapy?	Yes	No
Consider aspirin therapy (75-162 mg/d) as a <u>secondary prevention</u> in patients with type 1 or type 2 diabetes AND history of atherosclerotic cardiovascular disease Consider as <u>primary prevention</u> in those with diabetes, increased cardiovascular risk, after comprehensive discussion with patient (benefits vs risk of increased bleed risk) *Major CV risk factors include premature ASCVD, hypertension, dyslipidemia, smoking, CKD/albuminuria*		
Should I be on statin therapy?	Yes	No
≥40 years of age, CVD, or CVD risk factors include dyslipidemia, high blood pressure, smoking, and overweight/obesity, a family history of premature coronary disease, CKD, presence of albuminuria 20-39 years of age with additional ASCVD risk factors		

Vaccinations			
Annual Flu Vaccine	Yes	No	Date:
≥6 months of age			
COVID-19 Vaccine (*List below*)	Yes	No	Date(s):
Pfizer-BioNTech—age 6 months to 5 years old: administer 3-dose series Pfizer-BioNTech—age 5 or older: administer 2-dose series (21 days apart); booster(s) as needed Moderna—age 12 or older: administer 2-dose series (28 days apart); booster(s) for ≥18 years old as needed Janssen—age 18 or older: administer 1 dose; booster indicated 8 weeks after dose 1			

Vaccinations			
Pneumococcal Vaccine	**Yes**	**No**	**Date:**

Age 2-5: complete 4-dose series of pneumococcal conjugate vaccine 13 (PCV13) if not done by 15 months old

Age 6-18: administer 1 dose of pneumococcal polysaccharide vaccine 23 (PPSV23)

Age 19-64 with diabetes: if not previously vaccinated or unknown history, administer Prevnar 20 or PCV15 followed by PPSV23 a year after. *If previous PPSV23, may administer PCV15 or PCV20 a year after. **If previous PCV13, administer PPSV23 (8 weeks apart) then another dose PPSV23 (5 years apart).

Age ≥ 65 years of age: if not previously vaccinated or unknown history, should receive pneumococcal conjugate vaccine (PCV15 or PCV20). *If PCV15, dose of PPSV23 8 weeks (if immunocompromised) to 12 months after initial vaccination is recommended. **If PCV20, PPSV23 not indicated unless HCP deems necessary. Age ≥65 years of age: if previously vaccinated with PPSV23, should receive a follow-up ≥12 months with PCV13.

Hepatitis B Vaccination	**Yes**	**No**	

Age 19-59: administer hepatitis B vaccination (2- or 3-dose series) to unvaccinated adults with diabetes.

Age 60 or older and at increased risk for hepatitis B, then you and your provider may decide if needed.

DM Complications/Comorbidities Management				
	Major Complications/Comorbidities			
	History of ASCVD or High ASCVD Risks	**Heart Failure**	**Chronic Kidney Disease With Albuminuria**	**Chronic Kidney Disease Without Albuminuria**
First line	GLP-1 receptor agonists or SGLT-2 inhibitors	SGLT-2 inhibitors with proven benefits HFpEF: Jardiance HFrEF: Farxiga, Jardiance	+SGLT-2 inhibitors with primary evidence of reducing CKD +Invokana (if urine albumin excretion >300 mg/d) +Farxiga (adjunctive therapy if UACr >200 mg/g) Kerendia (finerenone) (may initiate if eGFR ≥25 mL/min/1.73 m²; must monitor potassium prior to initiation and during therapy)	SGLT-2 inhibitors with primary evidence of reducing CKD

DM Complications/Comorbidities Management				
	Major Complications/Comorbidities			
	History of ASCVD or High ASCVD Risks	**Heart Failure**	**Chronic Kidney Disease With Albuminuria**	**Chronic Kidney Disease Without Albuminuria**
If A1c above target despite one or other agents	Consider dual therapy: GLP-1RA and SGLT2-i		Consider dual therapy: GLP-1RA and SGLT2-i	Consider dual therapy: GLP-1RA and SGLT2-i
Third line	TZD			
Other agents to manage comorbidities	ACE-inhibitors or ARBs Aspirin Statins	*ACE-inhibitors or ARBs or ARNI *Beta-blockers (bisoprolol, carvedilol, metoprolol succinate) ± Loop diuretics for symptom management ± *MRAs *Titrate to target doses	ACE-inhibitors or ARBs ± Phosphate binders ± Iron supplementation or ESAs if anemia of CKD ± Vitamin D	ACE-inhibitors or ARBs ± Phosphate binders ± Iron supplementation or ESAs if anemia of CKD ± Vitamin D

Avoid the Need for Fasting Lab Work

Requiring fasting labs can delay care and may cause unnecessary risk to the patient. As mentioned in this case, the patient experienced hypoglycemia attempting to get fasting lab work on at least two occasions. Historically, fasting results were thought necessary to help guide glucose management. This is no longer the case as patients now provide us with fasting glucose readings via self-monitoring and with multiple data points. We no longer require fasting lipid levels either. Current guidelines emphasize intensity-based statin therapy as opposed to treating to LDL targets. Of note, our practice finds the use of nonfasting triglycerides to be useful in measuring insulin resistance.

Have Dedicated Diabetes-Only Visits

A person with diabetes lives with the condition for 8760 h/y. Devoting 1 to 2 h/y to clinical management should be a bare minimum. Yet, accomplishing this can be a real challenge in the primary care setting where people often present with multiple complaints or chronic conditions they want to address. If I have a patient who was originally scheduled for a diabetes recheck but presents with additional concerns, I will ask them which they want to focus on today Rather than try to address both issues, I may recommend that we focus on the patient's concern and reschedule their diabetes visit. I tell the patient that their concern and their diabetes management are both very important. Trying to address both in a single visit will result in neither getting the attention they deserve.

There are so many important points to review in diabetes care. Helping people develop treatment regimens, assisting with self-management plans, addressing fears and concerns, providing patient education, and promoting patient empowerment requires a significant time commitment. Being able to dedicate time to diabetes specifically is critical for patient success.

4. There are many tools available to help our patients with these regimens. Our patient is taking basal insulin and rapid-acting insulin. The rapid-acting insulin is provided with a carb ratio (for food to be ingested) and a correction scale for hyperglycemia. However, she is struggling with inconsistent results.

There are apps that can help a person calculate an insulin dose and smart pens that will do the same (Table 7.1). These do require an initial setup by the clinician but can be very helpful for the patient. A select list of apps is provided.[7] *Clinical Diabetes* (a journal of the ADA focused on practical information for primary care) published a special issue on Diabetes Technology in Primary Care in 2020, which is a great resource for those who want to learn more.[8]

The journal also included a patient page to log food, insulin, and glucose to help determine accuracy of carb count and correction scale. Handouts are shown below.

TABLE 7.1   Select List of Computer/Phone Apps That Help With Diabetes Management[7]

App Name	Platform	Tool	Cost (2022)
mySugr	Apple/Android	Glucose tracking	$19.99-399/y
iHealth Gluco-smart	Apple/Android	Glucose tracking	Free with system
One Drop	Apple/Android	Glucose tracking	17.99/mo
MyFitnessPal	Apple/Android	Lifestyle support	Free
CalorieKing	Apple	Lifestyle support	Free
Glucose Buddy	Apple	Lifestyle support	Basic: free

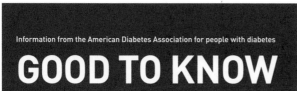

Information from the American Diabetes Association for people with diabetes

GOOD TO KNOW

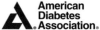

American Diabetes Association®

Making Sense of BGM Data for a Basal-Bolus Insulin User

DATE		Fasting or Pre-breakfast	Post-breakfast or Pre-lunch	Post-lunch or Pre-dinner	Post-dinner or Bedtime
	TIME				
	GLUCOSE				
	CARBS				
	INSULIN				
NOTES					

DATE		Fasting or Pre-breakfast	Post-breakfast or Pre-lunch	Post-lunch or Pre-dinner	Post-dinner or Bedtime
	TIME				
	GLUCOSE				
	CARBS				
	INSULIN				
NOTES					

DATE		Fasting or Pre-breakfast	Post-breakfast or Pre-lunch	Post-lunch or Pre-dinner	Post-dinner or Bedtime
	TIME				
	GLUCOSE				
	CARBS				
	INSULIN				
NOTES					

Standard fasting or pre-meal glucose target range:

80–130 mg/dL or custom range:

_____

Standard post-meal glucose target range:

80–180 mg/dL or custom range:

_____

When your fasting or pre-breakfast glucose is consistently high:
Consider eating fewer carbs with dinner. Consider being more active in the evening. If the glucose doesn't come down with your own efforts, discuss an adjustment of your insulin dose with your diabetes care team.

When your post-meal glucose is consistently high:
Consider eating fewer carbs with your meals. Discuss an adjustment of your insulin dose with your care team.

When you have frequent hypoglycemia:
Discuss an adjustment of your insulin dose with your care team.

Basal insulin name:
_____

Morning dose: _____units
Evening dose: _____units

Bolus insulin name:
_____

Dosing type: ☐ fixed dose with meals
☐ insulin-to-carb ratio
☐ correctional scale

Fixed dose	**Insulin-to-carb ratio**	**Correctional scale**
Breakfast dose: ___units	Breakfast dose: ___units/g	Add 1 unit of insulin
Lunch dose: ___units	Lunch dose: ___units/g	for every ___mg/dL
Dinner dose: ___units	Dinner dose: ___units/g	over ___mg/dL.

Always follow the instructions for taking your insulin provided to you by your health care team. Have a plan to treat hypoglycemia (glucose <70 mg/dL) and a plan for days when you are sick. Report all serious hypoglycemia.

This handout was written by Mansur E. Shomali and published in *Clinical Diabetes*, Vol. 38, issue 5, 2020. Copyright American Diabetes Association, Inc., 2020.

Making Sense of CGM Data for a Basal-Bolus Insulin User

	TIME IN RANGE	TIME BELOW RANGE	TIME ABOVE RANGE
Definition	The percentage of your readings between 70 and 180 mg/dL	The percentage of your readings <70 mg/dL (low) or <54 mg/dL (very low)	The percentage of your readings >180 mg/dL (high) or >250 mg/dL (very high)
Standard Target	>70%	<4% low; <1% very low	<25% high; <5% very high
Custom Target			
Your data/date			
Your data/date			
Your data/date			

- Before meals, use current glucose data and trend arrow in calculating insulin doses and deciding whether to deliver doses before or after eating.
- Two hours after meals, determine whether correctional insulin is needed.

- At bedtime, use current glucose data and trend arrow to decide whether corrective action is needed to prevent nighttime hypoglycemia or hyperglycemia.
- During and after exercise, monitor glucose every 15–30 minutes to prevent hypoglycemia.

- During sick days, monitor glucose levels at least every 4 hours. Vitamin C and aspirin may affect the accuracy of glucose readings with FreeStyle Libre and Medtronic CGM devices. (FreeStyle Libre 2 is not affected by aspirin.)

Medtronic	Dexcom	FreeStyle Libre	Trend Meaning	Glucose Value	Actions to Help You Stay or Get in Range
↑↑↑	↑↑		Glucose rising >3 mg/dL/min	High	▶ Take correctional insulin if you have not already done so in the past 2 hours. ▶ If you will eat, you can take your bolus insulin for your meal **before** you start eating; do not consume food, snacks, or drinks containing carbs until the trend arrow levels off.
↑↑	↑	↑	Glucose rising 2–3 mg/dL/min (>2 mg/dL/min for FreeStyle Libre)	In range	▶ Your glucose is fine right now but rising; check back in 15 minutes. ▶ If you will eat, you can take your bolus insulin for your meal **before** you start eating; do not consume food, snacks, or drinks containing carbs until the trend arrow levels off.
↑	↗	↗	Glucose rising 1–2 mg/dL/min	Low	▶ Your glucose is currently low but moving in the right direction; check back in 5 minutes. ▶ If you will eat, you can take your bolus insulin for your meal **after** you start eating; do not take your bolus until your glucose is out of the low range.
No arrow	→	→	Glucose changing slowly <1 mg/dL/min	High	▶ Take correctional insulin if you have not already done so in the past 2 hours. ▶ If you will eat, you can take your bolus insulin for your meal **before** you start eating; do not consume food, snacks, or drinks containing carbs until the trend arrow levels off.
				In range	▶ If you will eat, you can take your bolus insulin for your meal **before** you start eating.
				Low	▶ Your glucose is currently low; to correct it, consume fast-acting carbs (usually 4 oz of juice or 3–4 glucose tablets); check back in 5 minutes. ▶ If you will eat, you can take your bolus insulin for your meal **after** you start eating; do not take your bolus until your glucose is out of the low range.
↓	↘	↘	Glucose falling 1–2 mg/dL/min	High	▶ Your glucose is currently high but moving in the right direction; check back in 15 minutes. ▶ If you will eat, you can take your bolus insulin for your meal **after** you start eating; do not take your bolus until the trend arrow levels off.
↓↓	↓	↓	Glucose falling 2–3 mg/dL/min (>2 mg/dL/min for FreeStyle Libre)	In range	▶ Your glucose is fine right now but falling; check back in 5 minutes. ▶ If you will eat, you can take your bolus insulin for your meal **after** you start eating; do not take your bolus until the trend arrow levels off.
↓↓↓	↓↓		Glucose falling >3mg/dL/min	Low	▶ Your glucose is currently low; to correct it, consume fast-acting carbs (usually 8 oz of juice or 6–8 glucose tablets); check back in 5 minutes. ▶ If you will eat, you can take your bolus insulin for your meal **after** you start eating; do not take your bolus until your glucose is out of the low range.

Basal insulin name:
_____

Morning dose: _____ units
Evening dose: _____ units

Always follow the instructions for taking your insulin provided to you by your health care team. Have a plan to treat hypoglycemia (glucose <70 mg/dL) and a plan for days when you are sick. Report all serious hypoglycemia.

Bolus insulin name:
_____

Dosing type: ☐ fixed dose with meals
☐ insulin-to-carb ratio
☐ correctional scale

Fixed dose	**Insulin-to-carb ratio**	**Correctional scale***
Breakfast dose: ___units	Breakfast dose: ___units/g	Add 1 unit of insulin for every ___mg/dL over ___mg/dL.
Lunch dose: ___units	Lunch dose: ___units/g	
Dinner dose: ___units	Dinner dose: ___units/g	

*Some CGM users may adjust their insulin dose using the trend arrow. Discuss whether you should do this with your diabetes care team.

American Diabetes Association.

This handout was written by Mansur E. Shomali and published in *Clinical Diabetes*, Vol. 38, issue 5, 2020. Copyright American Diabetes Association, Inc., 2020.

Used with permission from American Diabetes Association (ADA). Making sense of BGM and CGM data for a Basal-Bolus insulin user. *Clin Diabetes*. 2020;38(5):501-502. https://doi.org/10.2337/cd20-pe05

Case Summary and Closing Points

Helping people manage their diabetes can be challenging. Fortunately, there is a plethora of tools that make it easier for both the person with diabetes and their health care team. Advances in diabetes technology have improved patients' ability to engage in self-management and enhanced clinicians' ability to guide care. Clinician knowledge of these tools and sharing them with your patients can really help support them in the day-to-day management.

References

1. Glooko mobile app. Accessed December 28, 2022. https://www.glooko.com/people-with-diabetes/
2. Tidepool Project. Tidepool App. Accessed December 28, 2022. https://www.tidepool.org/users
3. Whitley HP, Hanson C, Parton JM. Systematic diabetes screening using point-of-care HbA1c testing facilitates identification of prediabetes. *Ann Fam Med*. 2017;15(2):162-164.
4. Grieve R, Beech R, Vincent J, et al. Near patient testing in diabetes clinics: appraising the costs and outcomes. *Health Technol Assess*. 1999;3(15):1-74.
5. Miller CD, Barnes CS, Phillips LS, et al. Rapid A1c availability improves clinical decision-making in an urban primary care clinic. *Diabetes Care*. 2003;26(4):1158-1163.
6. Laurence CO, Gialamas A, Bubner T, et al. Patient satisfaction with point-of-care testing in general practice. *Br J Gen Pract*. 2010;60(572):e98-e104.
7. Doyle-Delgado K, Chamberlain JJ. Use of diabetes-related applications and digital health tools by people with diabetes and their health care clinician. Diabetes technology issue in primary care. *Clin Diabetes*. 2020;38(5)449-461.
8. Shomali ME. Diabetes technology issue in primary care. *Clin Diabetes*. 2020;38(5):417-502. https://diabetesjournals.org/clinical/issue/38/5

Case 2. Targeted Glucose Monitoring

"I do not understand why I am always normal at home but high in the office."

A 48-year-old man presents for a diabetes recheck. He was diagnosed with diabetes 6 years ago. He suspects he has had it longer, though, since he did not use to go to a doctor. Generally, he has been feeling well and reports that he does not typically "feel his diabetes." His morning glucose readings are usually around 100 mg/dL. He does not check his glucose during the day because he works with his hands, and they are not clean enough for him to poke his finger. By the time he gets home at night, all he has the energy to do is "kiss my wife, yell at my kids, eat, shower, and go to bed." He mentions that he hates having his glucose checked at his appointments because it is always high. He does not understand this because his readings are OK at home. He is "using the best meter" according to his pharmacist.

Med HX: type 2 diabetes, hypertension, dyslipidemia

Medications: metformin 1000 mg bid, insulin glargine 48 U/d, atorvastatin 40 mg daily, valsartan 160 mg daily

Allergies: sulfa—rash

Family Medical History: strong FH of type 2 diabetes

Social History: lives with his spouse. Two kids; ages 14 and 16. Works in landscaping. His wife packs a lunch for him each day. He gets hungry mid-day and often snacks on cakes or cookies.

Physical Exam: Ht. 5′7″, Wt. 187 lb, BMI 29.3, P 72, R 18, BP 122/78

GEN: obese male with truncal obesity in no distress

HEENT: normal including thyroid exam

CV: normal

RESP: normal

Extremities: normal peripheral pulses, normal sensation to monofilament exam

Labs: HbA1c 8.4%

Random glucose: 224 mg/dL (2 PM)

 CASE QUESTIONS

1. What is contributing to the mismatch between home glucose monitoring and his HbA1c? How should this be addressed?
2. How can he determine what his glucose is doing at work and overnight?
3. What does his targeted testing indicate?
4. What do you recommend for treatment for him?

 ANSWERS AND EXPLANATIONS

1. According to our patient, his fasting glucose is consistently ~100 mg/dL. If his glucose was in this range throughout the day, he would have an HbA1c of 6.0%. However, his HbA1c is 8.4%, which indicates a glucose of about 200 mg/dL. He is clearly having glucose excursions that need to be explained.

   The first step is to learn more about the patient's daily routine. What does he eat and drink? When does he eat his meals? What is the nature of his work?

   He reports that he wakes at 5:30 AM and typically has oatmeal for breakfast ("it is good for my cholesterol"). He often drives through his favorite fast-food restaurant on the way to work to get a breakfast sandwich and a latte. His work is physically demanding; he spends his days outdoors in the sun. His beverage of choice is Gatorade; he will drink several throughout the day. His lunchtime varies but is usually in the early afternoon. His wife packs his lunch. This usually includes a sandwich, fruit, and sometimes a snack cake. He will have another Gatorade and a snack cake later in the day if it is hot. He usually arrives home by 6 PM and eats dinner at 6:30 PM. Dinner usually consists of chicken or beef, potatoes, and a small salad. He used to check his glucose at bedtime. It was usually high. This created conflict with his wife, so he stopped checking at night.

   The patient is currently treating his diabetes with metformin and insulin glargine. Both are excellent medications, but they have a similar effect on glycemic control. They primarily impact fasting glucose levels. His fasting glucose is well-controlled. Based on his elevated HbA1c, his problem is not being able to adequately respond to his dietary intake. As a result, he is frequently hyperglycemic. He confirmed this via his bedtime readings.

Clearly, his dietary choices need to be addressed; he would benefit from working with a dietician. A discussion regarding the effects eating has on his glucose levels and how that differs from fasting glucose regulation may be useful. In addition, we should discuss an adjustment to his diabetes regimen to better address postprandial glucose elevations. Ideally, we would want him to begin postprandial testing. If he is not comfortable performing fingerstick glucose readings during the day, a CGM could be a better option.

This is also an important time to recognize the work he is doing—first AM glucose checks and his interest and involvement to figure out what is contributing to the inconsistencies in his readings. A study found that 1 in 6 patients who were performing self-monitoring of blood glucose (SMBG) were never acted on by the patient or clinician.[1]

2. This is a great time to implement "targeted" or "structured" glucose checks. This can be done in several ways.

   • The International Diabetes Federation (IDF) recommends intensive or focused glucose testing. This requires 5 to 7 glucose checks (fasting/prebreakfast, postbreakfast, prelunch, postlunch, predinner, postdinner, and bedtime) for 1 to 3 days while the patient is performing their usual activity and eating typical meals. This enables the clinician (and patient) to recognize glucose patterns. Postmeal tests are typically 90 to 120 minutes after eating.[2] While this approach is often used internationally, it has not been generally adopted in the United States.

   • Another option is "staggered checking."[3] With this approach, glucose is checked at different times for several days. For example, on Monday the glucose checks could be fasting and bedtime. Tuesday could be prebreakfast and postbreakfast, Wednesday—prelunch and postlunch, and Thursday—pre- and postdinner. This approach is less labor-intensive and less likely to disrupt an individual's routine. It yields similar data to the IDF approach. Importantly, it is a practical strategy for people for whom the rate-limiting factor for self-monitoring is the number of test strips their insurance covers each day.

   • We will sometimes ask patients to check glucose at bedtime and fasting to determine the bedtime to am difference (BeAM).[4] This can be informative in patients with fasting hyperglycemia and overnight hypoglycemia and can help differentiate Somogyi from Dawn phenomena.

   In this patient's case, it appears that the treatments focused on controlling fasting glucose are working. Since we are confident about his fasting glucose levels, I would ask him to stop checking in the morning and begin checking before and after dinner. This allows him to get some sense of what happens to his glucose during the workday. His predinner readings should reflect his daytime glucose control and may be acceptable because he is very physically active at work. Because of this, it is possible that he does not need medications to manage his glucose after breakfast and lunch. Perhaps more importantly, with his postdinner check, we can see what his glucose excursion is with dinner. Based on his HbA1c and his prior testing, we expect his glucose levels will be high. If his schedule allows obtaining pre- and postlunch readings on a nonworkday, this would also be useful.

3. With the encouragement of his spouse, he agreed to do checks at other times of the day but was adamant that he could not test at work. His plan was to check each morning and night on workdays, and on weekends he agreed to check before lunch, and either after lunch or before dinner. His glucose readings are listed below.

	Fasting/ PreBreakfast	Prelunch	Predinner	Postdinner	Bedtime
Monday	112			280	
Tuesday	120			230	242
Wednesday	108			188	
Thursday	111				212
Friday	130		216		
Saturday		190	230		
Sunday		168	203		

4. We clearly see from his structured glucose monitoring that he has postprandial hyperglycemia. This can be accomplished several ways. He can continue to reduce his snacking and carbohydrates at meals and snacks. He could also add a medication that addresses postprandial hyperglycemia. These could include a DPP-4 inhibitor, acarbose, a GLP-1RA, or mealtime insulin.

Case Summary and Closing Points

The management of diabetes can be a mystery to many patients. Often the only insight for many people is their home glucose readings and periodic HbA1c readings. Unfortunately, this may not provide enough context to determine best management practices for their diabetes. As we saw in this case, those readings may not match. The use of targeted glucose monitoring provides a much richer description of how a person's daily activities affect glucose levels. Further, this provided an opportunity to educate the patient on how to adjust daily lifestyle habits and medications to help him meet the glucose goals.

References

1. Grant RW, Huang ES, Wexler DJ, et al. Patients who self-monitor blood glucose and their unused testing results. *Am J Manag Care*. 2015;21(2):e119-e129.
2. IDF SMBG Guidelines. Accessed December 28, 2022. https://www.idf.org/e-library/guidelines/85-self-monitoring-of-blood-glucose-in-non-insulin-treated-type-2-diabetes.html
3. Logan AD, Jones J, Kuritzky L. Structured blood glucose monitoring in primary care: a practical, evidence-based approach. *Clin Diabetes*. 2020;38(5):421-428. doi:10.2337/cd20-0045
4. Stuhr A, Zisman A, Morales F, Stewart J, Vlajnic A, Zhou R. BeAM value: an indicator of the need to initiate and intensify prandial therapy in patients with type 2 diabetes mellitus receiving basal insulin. *BMJ Open Diabetes Res Care*. 2016;4(1):e000171. doi:10.1136/bmjdrc-2015-000171

Case 3. Introducing Glucose Sensors

"Can I shower with this thing?"

A 28-year-old woman presents for her diabetes recheck. You met her in the last chapter when she was asking about the risk of her child getting diabetes Chapter 6 (case 4). She and her partner are ready to start a family, and she wants help preparing for a safe pregnancy. As you may recall, she was experiencing a fair number of hypoglycemic episodes.

She considered an insulin pump in the past but did not want something connected to her all the time. She described wearing a pump as attaching "a big shiny diabetes billboard" to herself. At your urging, she did some research online about different devices to improve diabetes management. At this point, she is ready to consider using a CGM to get early warnings about her lows. She presents for more information and specifically wants to know if she wears one, if can she shower and exercise and do her normal activities.

Med HX: type 1 diabetes (14 years), mild background retinopathy

Medications: insulin detemir 32 units each morning, insulin aspart 1:7 carb ratio for breakfast, 1:8 units for lunch and dinner, correction factor 1:25 above 125 mg/dL

Allergies: none

Family Medical History: dad with vitiligo, mom with hypothyroidism

Social History: lives with a partner; never was pregnant; works as a web designer; no tobacco use; drinks wine occasionally; walks at work some days at lunch

Physical Exam: Ht. 5′6″, 148 lb, BMI 23.8, P 70, R 15, BP 130/72

GEN: in no distress

HEENT: normal including thyroid exam

CV: normal

RESP: normal

Skin: injection sites largely intact but some lipohypertrophy noted on both deltoid areas

Extremities: normal pulses, good skin care, no loss of sensation to monofilament

Home glucose readings: checks 6 to 10 times per day; tries to get ahead of the highs but still having some lows; especially if she corrects too much or if she eats less than she thinks she is going to eat

Labs: HbA1c 6.4%

CASE QUESTIONS

1. What are the currently available continuous glucose monitors (CGM)?
2. Who is a good candidate for a CGM?
3. How can we help a person choose a CGM?
4. What is the process of ordering a CGM?
5. How did this patient do on a CGM?

 ANSWERS AND EXPLANATIONS

1. This patient is actively engaged in her diabetes management. She is using her meter to determine her insulin doses and to monitor her blood sugar. The use of a CGM will help reduce her workload and provide her with more information. She will be better able to track her glucose levels than she could with fingerstick glucose readings. She will also have access to overnight information she was not able to get previously. Choosing a CGM that provides alerts when glucose levels are too high or low will provide an additional layer of safety.

There are several CGM systems available. They are summarized in Table 7.2. Remember, helping a patient review their options helps promote shared decision-making and engenders trust. It is important for patients to know that the clinician's goal is to help meet their needs. Letting the patient review the choices allows for shared decision-making and can help the patient meet her needs.

There are two broad categories of CGM systems. The first include personal systems. These are prescribed for the patient and are typically placed by the patient. They are intended for long-term use. Data are visible and actionable for the patient at the time of wear. These devices are typically covered by most insurers for patients who are on insulin, but coverage can vary for other patients. There are several different brands of personal CGM systems. They differ in how often their sensors need to be replaced, the need for calibration, whether they interface with other devices (pumps), and whether data can be shared or accessed online (Table 7.2). The manufacturers of these devices provide training videos to help people start and manage the devices.[1-3]

The second category of CGM devices is the Professional (Pro) units. These are typically practice-owned and are placed on patients in the office—much like a Holter monitor. Pro systems are used for a limited period to obtain additional information to help determine treatment decisions. Patients return them at the end of the CGM wear when the device is downloaded, and the data are reviewed by the clinician (Table 7.3).

To answer our patient's first question, all CGM devices are water resistant. She can bathe, shower, exercise, and play sports with these tools. There are some limitations; they should not be submersed for extended periods of time, for example in a hot tub or while swimming.

She should know that these sensors should be removed before a person has a CT scan, an MRI, or enters a magnetic device.

It is important to inform her that several commonly used substances can cause inaccurate readings, depending on which device is being used.[4]

The **Freestyle system** has the following warnings:

TABLE 7.2   Currently Available Personal CGM Systems

CGM System	Sensor Life	Calibration Needed	Intermittently Scanned or Real Time Continuous	Alarms for High and Low	Does Reader/ Screen Show Trends?	Compatible to Smart Device	Data Sharing With Others?
Abbott Freestyle 14 day Libre	14 days	No	Intermittently scanned	No	Yes	Yes	Yes
Abbott Freestyle Libre 2	14 days	No	Real time	Yes	Yes	Yes	Yes
Abbott Freestyle Libre 3	14 days	No	Real time	Yes	Yes	Yes	Yes
Dexcom G6	10 days	No	Real time	Yes	Yes	Yes	Yes
Medtronic Guardian Connect	7 days	Yes, every 12 hours	Real time	Yes	Yes	Yes	Yes
Senseonics Eversense	Up to 90 days	Yes, every 12 hours	Real time	Yes	Yes	Yes	Yes

TABLE 7.3 Currently Available CGM Pro Systems			
CGM System	**Sensor Life (days)**	**Calibration Needed**	**Blinded**
Abbott Freestyle Pro	14	No	Yes
Dexcom G6 Pro	10	No	Optional
Medtronic iPro 2	7	Yes	Yes

- Taking ascorbic acid (vitamin C) while wearing a Libre sensor may cause elevated glucose readings.
- Taking salicylic acid, either orally or used topically, may slightly lower sensor glucose readings.

In both situations, the degree of error is dependent on the amount of interfering substance present in the body.[4]

The **DEXCOM system** has the following warning[5]:

- Taking a higher than the maximum dose of acetaminophen (eg, > 1 g every 6 hours in adults) may falsely raise sensor glucose readings. This effect appears to be more significant in women than men.[2]

The **Medtronic system** has the following warning[6]:

- Taking medications containing acetaminophen while wearing the sensor may falsely raise sensor glucose readings. The level of inaccuracy depends on the amount of acetaminophen active in the body and may be different for each person.[3]

This is an important time to remind her that if she is uncertain about the accuracy of any CGM readings she should always use glucose meter readings to verify her glucose level before making therapy decisions.

2. CGM devices could benefit any patient who desires more information about their glucose control. They enable the wearer to see how their daily activities affect their glucose levels. They are a wonderful resource for the provider to help guide medication management; they are very helpful when troubleshooting hyperglycemia and hypoglycemia. They can be useful tools for patients to help drive behavior change (for example, our first patient in this chapter). While we can offer Pro units to most patients, the reality is that payors dictate who can receive personal devices. Most often, patients need to be using insulin for insurance to cover a device. Having said this, there is a rationale to provide a "trial run" of a device. This can sometimes provide the necessary documentation of glucose instability required to obtain authorization for the device.

   Our patient is an ideal candidate for a CGM. She is on a complex insulin regimen that includes both basal and bolus insulin based on carbohydrate counting. She performs multiple checks per day. Having a CGM would eliminate the need for her to perform fingerstick glucose readings. It would also provide many more data points both you and she can use to guide her insulin dosing. She is also having a lot of lows, so she would really benefit from a system that shows trends and has alarms.

It would be worth asking her if she has a preference regarding the need to calibrate a CGM device with fingerstick glucose readings. We will also want to know if she wants to share her data. This information will help us identify the best unit to meet her needs.

3. Most insurers cover the range of CGM devices, so the choice can really be individualized.

    I find the best practice is to show the patient all of the devices available. I like them to see the size of the sensors, and how they are applied. I also like to review the options each system has for monitoring glucose levels. Most patients like the ability to use their smartphone to monitor their glucose. Giving patients the opportunity to learn more about their choices can improve patient satisfaction with CGM. The https://diabeteswise.org/#/ website provides an unbiased "consumer reports" review of the CGM devices.[7] Many patients will have researched their options in advance and know what they want when they come into the office there is also a version of this website for clinicians at: https://pro.diabeteswise.org/#/.[8]

    If your office has access to the Pro versions of these units or samples of the personal CGM devices, you might offer the patient a device to try for a short period of time. This can be very helpful if you have a patient who is uncertain about using a CGM, or if they are unsure which unit they prefer.

4. For most devices, ordering a CGM system is as simple as "writing" a prescription. Most primary care clinician will likely utilize either the Dexcom or Abbott devices. If you are new to using CGMs, it may be worthwhile to reach out to your local sales representatives. They can help improve your familiarity with the different units. There are several components that will need to be prescribed depending on which system you and your patient choose. These devices are obtained at the patient's pharmacy.

Unfortunately, regardless of which device is ordered, there may be a need for prior authorization. This will quickly become apparent depending on where you practice and your payor mix.

Medicaid coverage for CGM devices varies by state. CGM devices are covered under Medicare Part-B. Medicare coverage criteria as of the writing of this text are the following:

- The patient has diabetes;
- The patient is insulin-treated with three or more daily administrations of insulin or a continuous subcutaneous insulin infusion (CSII) pump;
- The patient's insulin treatment regimen requires frequent adjustments based on BGM or CGM testing results;
- Within 6 months prior to ordering the CGM, the patient had an in-person visit with the treating practitioner to evaluate their diabetes control and determine that the above criteria have been met; and
- Every 6 months following the initial prescription of the CGM, the patient has an in-person visit with the treating practitioner to assess adherence to their CGM regimen and diabetes treatment plan.

It is important to note that Medtronic's and Sensonics' devices differ in that they are considered durable medical equipment, and as such are obtained from equipment suppliers as opposed to pharmacies (Dexcom and Freestyle Libre products).

If you are new to using CGM, it may be worth talking to your sales representative for details on each device to get help starting people on this system. After you have started three people, you will probably find the process to be quite easy.

5. This patient chose the 10-day DEXCOM sensor. She liked the fact that it did not need to be calibrated. She would have liked a sensor that lasted longer than 10 days; however, she was also considering an insulin pump and wanted to have a CGM that was compatible.

She set the sensor alarms for 80 mg/dL and 180 mg/dL. At first, the alarms sounded frequently. She found the corrective actions she required were smaller since she could quickly identify glucose highs and lows. As a result, her glucose levels did not swing up and down as much. With the data, she and I were able to adjust her mealtime ratios and reduce the frequency of her lows. She found the CGM to be much less bothersome than she thought it would be. She is happy knowing that with the CGM she can prevent hyperglycemic and hypoglycemic emergencies. She is now starting to look at choices for an insulin pump.

Case Summary and Closing Points

There have been amazing advances in diabetes technology. Continuous glucose monitoring systems have become more widely available, and as a result, their use has increased considerably. They are valuable tools for both the patient and the health care clinician to help improve glucose control. The reports from CGM devices provide important information on the patient's lived experience with diabetes. Personal CGM systems are typically covered for people who are taking insulin. Professional CGM units are a great introduction to these devices and are covered for most people with diabetes. There are many options; doing shared decision-making with the patient will increase patient use and satisfaction.

References

1. Abbott Libre tutorial videos. Accessed December 28, 2022. https://www.freestylelibre.us/support/overview.html?gclid=Cj0KCQjwiYL3BRDVARIsAF9E4Gd5brJCz3iSgVEp4uUUckLSUc8pZcawKg_YiF5jg_k3Xs9_Je9PHYEaArGuEALw_wcB
2. Dexcom training videos. Accessed December 28, 2022. https://www.dexcom.com/training-videos
3. Medtronic video libraryoref. Accessed December 28, 2022. https://www.medtronicdiabetes.com/customer-support/guardian-connect-system-support
4. Freestyle interference. Accessed December 28, 2022. https://www.freestyle.abbott/us-en/safety-information.html
5. Dexcom interference. Accessed December 28, 2022. www.dexcom.com/interference
6. *Medtronic safety warnings.* Accessed December 28, 2022. https://www.medtronic.com/us-en/healthcare-professionals/products/diabetes/indications-safety-warnings.html
7. Diabeteswise.org. Accessed December 28, 2022. https://diabeteswise.org/#/
8. ProDiabeteswise.org. Accessed December 28, 2022. https://pro.diabeteswise.org/#/

Case 4. **Benefits of Glucose Sensing**

"Now I can see what I need to do."

A 50-year-old man presents to establish care. His brother is the gentleman from Case 2 in this chapter. "My brother said I should see you. He said, "you know your stuff." He has had diabetes for 8 years. His last doctor told him his blood sugar was too high but did not tell him why or what to do about it. "My brother said I should try one of those sensor things." He suspects his diabetes is not very well controlled. He has some tingling in his feet that his last doctor said was from his diabetes. His eye doctor told him he has some diabetes in his eyes. Lately, he has had to urinate all the time and has been thirstier. His wife says this is from his sugar. He only checks his blood sugar in the morning several times a week. His readings are usually around 160 mg/dL. He stopped checking during the day and at night because his readings were always high. You offer to monitor him with a Pro CGM, and he agrees.

Med HX: type 2 diabetes, hypertension, dyslipidemia, diabetic neuropathy, diabetic retinopathy

Medications: metformin 1000 mg bid, insulin detemir 40 units daily, sitagliptin 50 mg daily, atorvastatin 40 mg daily, olmesartan 40 mg daily

Allergies: none

Family Medical History: strong FH of type 2 diabetes

Social History: lives with his spouse. Two kids—ages 20 and 24; works in landscaping

Physical Exam: Ht. 5'7", Wt. 197 lb, BMI 30.9, P 66, R 15, BP 132/74

GEN: obese male with truncal obesity in no distress

HEENT: normal including thyroid exam

CV: normal

RESP: normal

Extremities: normal peripheral pulses, decreased sensation to monofilament and vibration

Labs: HbA1c 10%

Random glucose: 244 mg/dL (4:30 PM)

CGM #1:

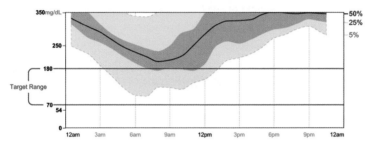

% Time CGM is Active	65%

Ranges And Targets For	Type 1 or Type 2 Diabetes
Glucose Ranges Target Range 70-180 mg/dL	**Targets % of Readings (Time/Day)** Greater than 70% (16h 48min)
Below 70 mg/dL	Less than 4% (58min)
Below 54 mg/dL	Less than 1% (14min)
Above 180 mg/dL	Less than 25% (6h)
Above 250 mg/dL	Less than 5% (1h 12min)
Each 5% increase in time in range (70-180 mg/dL) is clinically beneficial.	

Average Glucose	284 mg/dL
Glucose Management Indicator (GMI)	10.1%
Glucose Variability	29.5%
Defined as percent coefficient of variation (%CV); target ≤36%	

Very High >250 mg/dL	**63%**	(15h 7min)
High 181 - 250 mg/dL	**27%**	(6h 29min)
Target Range 70 - 180 mg/dL	**10%**	(2h 24min)
Low 54 - 69 mg/dL	**0%**	(0min)
Very Low <54 mg/dL	**0%**	(0min)

AMBULATORY GLUCOSE PROFILE (AGP)

AGP is a summary of glucose values from the report period, with median (50%) and other percentiles shown as if occurring in a single day.

[Graph: Ambulatory Glucose Profile showing glucose values across 24 hours from 12am to 12am, with y-axis marks at 350mg/dL, 250, 180, 70, 54, and 0. Percentile bands marked 50%, 25%, 5%. Target Range indicated between 70 and 180.]

 CASE QUESTIONS

1. What do you notice on his CGM report?
2. What treatments should you recommend?
3. How do you get CGM reports in your office?
4. How do you interpret CGM report data?
5. How do you get paid for placing CGMs and reading the reports?

 ANSWERS AND EXPLANATIONS

1. His CGM report is very telling. He indeed wakes up with a reading close to 180 mg/dL. Afterward, his glucose progressively increases to its peak reading of 350 mg/dL at 6:00 PM where it plateaus until midnight. His glucose decreases significantly overnight.

   At our follow-up, the patient and I reviewed his sensor report, and I asked him to walk me through his daily activities. He typically gets up around 7:00 AM and has a bowl of cereal. He and his brother drive through for a breakfast sandwich and some coffee on the way to work. They also usually pick up some snack cakes and Gatorade. He gets hungry mid-morning and mid-afternoon, so he snacks. At 6:00 PM he returns home and has whatever his wife has made for dinner. Dinner is his biggest meal of the day. "My wife is a really good cook!"

2. He has already started the treatment process. He has stopped (or at least reduced) his intake of sweetened beverages at work. Despite this, his numbers are still climbing while snacking during the workday. The goal here is to focus on treatments that will help him reduce postmeal hyperglycemia. Options include a DPP-4 inhibitor, a GLP-1RA, acarbose, and mealtime insulin. The patient is not interested in taking any medications that are dosed more than once a day. This excludes acarbose and mealtime insulin. Based on his current readings and keeping in mind an agreed A1c goal of <7.0%, we determine that he needs at least a 2.0% A1c reduction. He will likely be more successful with a GLP-1RA. He also likes the idea of being able to take the medication once weekly.

He starts a once-weekly GLP-1RA. This is effective in limiting his postprandial hyperglycemia, but he starts having some first AM hypoglycemia. He is able to reduce his insulin dose and achieve stable control. With the use of the CGM, he was really surprised to be able to see his glucose over the course of the day and now he really understands what he needs to do.

CGM #2:

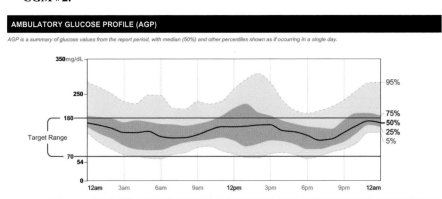

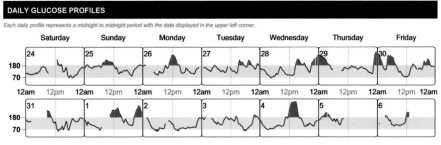

Source: Battelino, Tadej, et al. "Clinical Targets for Continuous Glucose Monitoring Data Interpretation: Recommendations From the International Consensus on Time in Range." Diabetes Care, American Diabetes Association, 7 June 2019, https://doi.org/10.2337/dci19-0028.

3. Each of the CGM devices comes with supportive software that can be utilized by the patient or the clinician. There are a couple of ways to access the data. Some offices have an online account with either the company or a service such as Glooko or Tidepool. With these programs, if the patient chooses to share their data (or gives "permission to view") clinicians can retrieve a report on a computer where it can be reviewed by the patient and clinician together. The other option is to

ask your office staff (usually the medical assistant or front office personnel) to download data as part of the check-in procedure. The report can then be printed or shared with the clinician to review on a computer. Finally, some patients upload data before the appointment and bring a printout to the office visit.

4. The first time you review a CGM report, you may find it overwhelming. Do not be discouraged. Data interpretation is easy to learn with a systematic approach and a little practice.

See the sample CGM report below (not from this patient).

Steps to CGM Download Interpretation[1]

Step 1: Confirm that you have adequate data to review. Seventy-two hours of continuous data are considered the minimum.

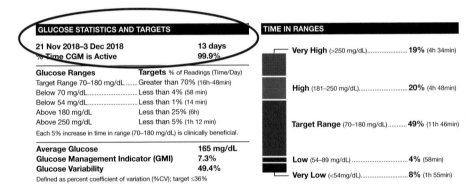

Step 2: Add in meal schedule and insulin dosing as relevant.

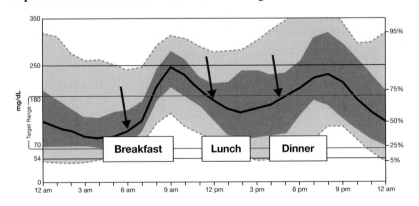

Step 3: Ask the patient what they see in terms of identifying highs and lows on the download report. This allows them to interpret without judgment.

Step 4: Identify the hypoglycemic episodes and explore the etiology.

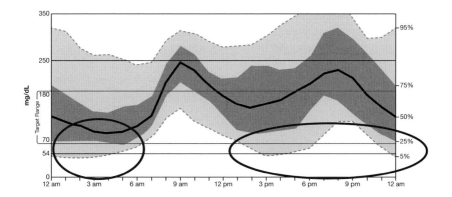

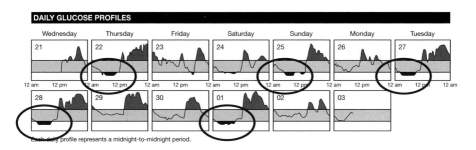

Step 5: Identify hyperglycemic episodes and explore etiology.

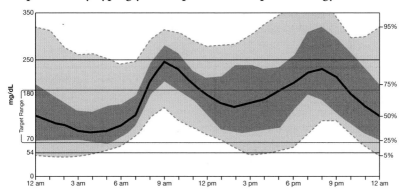

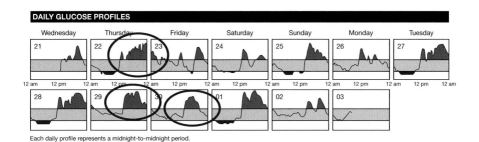

I would like to highlight that for this patient we did not identify the hyperglyce-mic reactions post hypoglycemia as an independent problem. We had to focus on the hypoglycemia first. The rebound hyperglycemia was a response to the hypoglycemia episode.

Step 6: Review summative data from the Ambulatory Glucose Profile including the Glucose Management Indicator (GMI) and Time in Range (TIR).

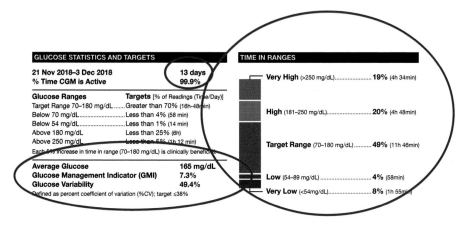

Step 7: Discuss treatment recommendations based on findings.

5. As mentioned earlier in the chapter, most insurances pay for professional CGM application and interpretation. Personal CGMs are usually covered in people who are on insulin and were doing frequent fingerstick glucose monitoring.

    Below is a summary of the billing codes and estimated payment for placing a personal CGM in the office (95,249), placing the professional CGM in the office (95,250) and the interpretation of the CGM device (95,251). Payment of a CGM is covered under the following circumstances: there is at least 72 hours of readable data, the clinician reports the main metrics in the ambulatory glucose profile (time warn, the time in range, above and below range, and glucose variability).

Case Summary and Closing Points

For this patient, allowing him to "see how his diabetes works" made all the dif-ference. Once he could see his patterns for himself, he felt empowered to make the necessary changes. He understood that he could control his diabetes instead of being controlled by it. Working in partnership, we decided on reasonable life-style behavior changes, modifications to his medication to reduce his postprandial hyperglycemia, and adjustments to his basal insulin dose to reduce risk of noctur-nal hypoglycemia. Helping a patient obtain a CGM and interpreting the data from

CGMs can be daunting at first, but the process does get easier over time and will, eventually, save you time.

Reference

1. Kruger DF, Edelman SV, Hinnen DA, Parkin CG. Reference guide for integrating continuous glucose monitoring into clinical practice. *Diabetes Educ.* 2019;45(1_suppl):3S-20S. doi:10.1177/0145721718818066

Case 5.   Drawbacks of Glucose Sensing

"I cannot do this anymore"

A 68-year-old woman presents for a diabetes recheck. She was initially diagnosed with type 2 diabetes 4 years ago, but 1 year ago she went into diabetic ketoacidosis (DKA) and found out that she had LADA (latent autoimmune diabetes of the adult), not type 2 diabetes.

At the last visit, she reported having a lot of unpredictable glucose readings. She could not understand what was making her glucose levels bounce so much. When offered a continuous glucose sensor, she said, "I am not sure. I do not even have a cell phone." With reassurance from the medical team and her spouse, she agreed to try it.

Med HX: type 1 diabetes, hypertension, generalized anxiety disorder

Medications: insulin glargine 18 units in the AM and 10 units in the PM, insulin lispro 4 units for a small meal and 6 units for a larger meal, atorvastatin 40 mg daily, metoprolol tartrate 50 mg bid

Allergies: none

Family Medical History: she was adopted and does not know her FH

Social History: lives with his spouse; no children, retired teacher

Physical Exam: Ht. 5′5″, Wt. 132 lb, BMI 22, P 92, R 20, BP 120/72

GEN: anxious but well female

HEENT: normal including thyroid exam

CV: normal

RESP: normal

Extremities: normal peripheral pulses, normal sensation to monofilament exam

Labs: HbA1c 7.0%

CGM report:

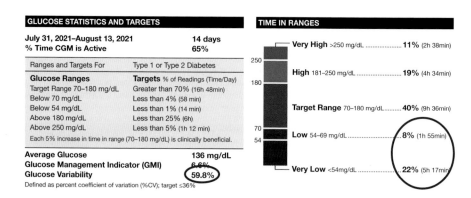

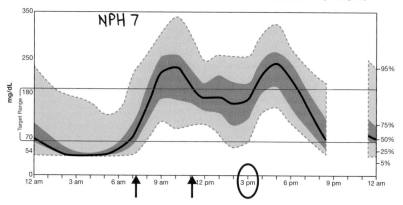

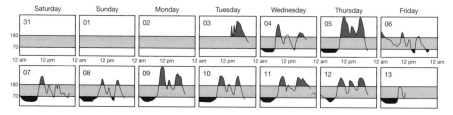

CASE QUESTIONS

1. What do you notice on the CGM report?
2. What questions do you have for the patient?
3. What treatments should you recommend?

ANSWERS AND EXPLANATIONS

1. This patient has a lot of extreme glucose variability. This is represented by the sharp peaks and valleys as seen on her sensor report. This is not only dangerous for the short- and long-term health of this patient; it feels really bad for the patient to experience this variability.

2. Start by asking the patient what they think about wearing the sensor. Is it something that they would like to have as a tool for their diabetes management? This patient said the sensor was terrible. She found it very stressful. Every time the glucose started to climb, she would get upset and start to worry, which seemed to make it climb higher. Then she would take some insulin, crash, and go too low. She reports that she can handle the lows most of the time. But she feels helpless against the relentless climb to hyperglycemia. The alarms from the device startled and scared her.

   She also reports concern that sometimes she did not feel the way she expected to, based on the CGM reading. The readings she finds could be 10 mg/dL different, and she was worried that it was not accurate.

3. Clearly, the amount of information for this patient was too overwhelming to be actionable. The information gained from CGM is intended to reveal general trends. The trend arrows are very important in terms of being able to anticipate changes. That being said, patients should allow enough time for their actions to affect their blood glucose.

   There are many things that can affect glucose other than food and insulin, particularly in people with type 1 diabetes. This is an important thing to remind people who are trying to understand all of the glucose changes they are experiencing. The glucose variability can also be a self-fulfilling cycle. The glucose starts to go up, and the person gets stressed, and this makes the glucose rise further.

Case Summary and Closing Points

While technology has improved the lives of many people with diabetes, it is not for everyone. It is important to engage your patient in the decision of what technology tools will work for them and which ones will not. For some people, the burden of managing another device or feeling like they need to respond to every change in glucose may be too much for them.

Case 6. Introduction to Insulin Pumps

"How do they implant that thing?"

A 22-year-old man presents for a diabetes recheck. He was diagnosed at age 10 years when he presented in DKA. He has had long periods when he felt that things were going well with his diabetes management. He has always used multiple daily doses of subcutaneous insulin as his treatment. He relates that he does not want to rely on a machine to manage his diabetes.

He recently moved to the area. He has a new friend who has diabetes and uses an insulin pump. His friend loves his pump and recommends that the patient discuss this option with his clinician.

Med HX: type 1 diabetes

Medications: insulin glargine 18 U/d, insulin lispro 1:10 carb ratio, and 1 per 50 above 100 correction factor

Allergies: shrimp—rash and itching

Family Medical History: none

Social History: none

Physical Exam: Ht. 5'9", Wt. 157 lb, BMI 23.2, P 72, R 12, BP 118/64

GEN: healthy male obesity in no distress

HEENT: normal including thyroid exam

CV: normal

RESP: normal

Extremities: normal peripheral pulses, normal sensation to monofilament exam

Labs:

Code	Description	Who Can Place and Initiate Sensor	Who Can Bill for Service	Medicare Physician Fee schedule	Medicare Outpatient Diabetes cente	Private Payor
95249	Ambulatory initiation of CGM of interstitial tissue fluid via a subcutaneous sensor for a minimum of 72 h; patient-owned equipment, sensor placement, hook-up, calibration of monitor, patient training, and printout of recording. The code requires the patient to bring the data receiver into the clinician office where the entire process is performed.	RN, PharmD/ RPh, RD, CDE, or MA within their scope of practice	Only MD/ DO, NP, PA, and CNS can bill for services associated with this code	44.80	44.80	~$132

Code	Description	Who Can Place and Initiate Sensor	Who Can Bill for Service	Medicare Physician Fee schedule	Medicare Outpatient Diabetes cente	Private Payor
95250	Ambulatory CGM of interstitial tissue fluid via a subcutaneous sensor for a minimum of 72 h; clinician-owned equipment, sensor placement, hook-up, calibration of monitor, patient training, removal of sensor, and printout of recording.	RN, PharmD/ RPh, RD, CDE, or MA within their scope of practice	Only MD/ DO, NP, PA, and CNS can bill for services associated with this code	~$156	~$122.63	~$300
95251	This code is used and reported to insurers when clinicians perform an analysis, interpretation, and report on a minimum of 72 h of CGM data. The analysis, interpretation, and report may be done with data from patient-owned or clinician-owned CGM device. Importantly, the analysis, interpretation, and report are distinct from an E/M service and does not include an assessment of the patient or indicate a plan of care for the patient.	N/A	Only MD/ DO, NP, PA, and CNS can bill for services associated with this code	~$36	Paid under physician fee schedule	~$89

Labs	Value	Reference Range
C-peptide	<0.01	0.78-1.89 ng/mL (fasting)
Islet cell antibody screen	Positive	Negative
GAD antibodies	62	<5 IU/mL

Lipid Panel	Value	Reference Range
Cholesterol, total	176	125-200 mg/dL
Triglycerides	80	<150 mg/dL
LDL (calculated)	91	<130 mg/dL
HDL cholesterol	65	>40 mg/dL men; >50 women
Non-HDL cholesterol	106	<130

CASE QUESTIONS

1. Who is eligible to use an insulin pump?
2. What are the different types of pumps?
3. How do you help this patient decide between devices?

 ANSWERS AND EXPLANATIONS

1. Currently, many insurance plans offer insulin pump therapy coverage for people with type 1 diabetes, provided that they meet the following three criteria:
   1. They are insulinopenic (as measured by a low C-peptide).
   2. They have completed diabetes education including carb counting training.
   3. They are practicing active diabetes management that includes multiple daily doses of insulin injections and frequent glucose monitoring used to adjust the insulin dose.

   It is common for insurance companies to request records of the above including lab results, glucose logs, and a note from the health care professional.

   Some insurers will also cover this benefit for people with type 2 diabetes who meet the second and third criteria. It should be noted that some people with longstanding type 2 diabetes can also become insulinopenic.

2. There are several insulin pumps available at this time and more will likely be available in the future.[1-3] To be able to understand how the pumps vary, I have highlighted some of the differences below.

Insulin Pump Alone

All of the insulin pumps can stand alone without the use of a continuous glucose sensor. The pumps deliver insulin based upon previously determined settings. In some respect they are "expensive syringes," but there are several features that really improve safety and convenience for the person with diabetes. For example, insulin pumps can accommodate multiple basal pattern settings. Maybe a person will need less insulin on the weekends than on weekdays because they are much more active on weekends. Insulin basal rates can vary over the course of the day. With an insulin pump, you can run a higher basal rate first thing in the most when insulin resistance is highest and run a lower basal rate in the middle of the night when insulin sensitivity (and risk of hypoglycemia) is greatest.

The other major feature of insulin pumps is the ability to help patients with the math needed for mealtime and correction insulin. Earlier in Chapter 4, we demonstrated how to calculate mealtime and correction doses. People on insulin pumps can enter the number of carbs they are about to eat and the current glucose, and the pump will calculate how much insulin they should take. This is made possible by preloading the carb ratio, the correction factor, and the target blood glucose.

The pump can also help reduce a person's risk of dropping low by calculating a smaller dose of insulin when the current glucose level is below the target range. This is termed reverse correction.

One final feature that makes insulin pumps safer is the ability to limit "stacking insulin." When a person with diabetes takes a correction dose of insulin for hyperglycemia, they should wait for the insulin to take effect. However, sometimes people become impatient, or the glucose does not respond quickly enough, and the person takes another dose of insulin to correct for the hyperglycemic episode. If this is administered before the full effects of the previous dose are gone, the person runs the risk of significant hypoglycemia from "stacking their insulin." Insulin pumps can prevent this by indicating how much insulin is still active from a previous dose. The pump-user can then adjust the current dose to prevent stacking.

Sensor-Augmented Insulin Pump

These pumps have all of the above features with the addition of a continuous glucose sensor that is communicating with the pump, thus providing additional safety features. Most important is the pump shut off when glucose is low. These pumps will sound an alarm when glucose is dropping too low. And, if the glucose gets to 70 mg/dL, the pump will suspend itself automatically to protect from more severe hypoglycemia.

Hybrid Closed Loop Pump[4-6]

These pumps have all the above features with the added ability to utilize current and projected sensor data to modify a dose of insulin. In short, the sensors continuously monitor glucose levels and send data to the pump to make minor adjustments to insulin delivery rate. This helps to maintain glucose levels within the desired range. The one thing these systems are unable to do is determine how to safely cover the insulin needs for meals. Instead, it is recommended that the pump-user enter each food intake and carb amount into the pump to more effectively deliver a bolus to cover intake.

Looping/DIY Systems[6-8]

These are novel systems used by people with diabetes. These systems have even greater interactivity between the sensor and the insulin pump. They often use old "hacked" pumps and a device that links the pump to the sensor and insulin algorithm—such as a Riley link device. While they are not approved by the FDA, they have been shown to be incredibly effective systems.

Another point of differentiation is whether the pump is "tubeless" or has catheter tubing.

The most common "tubed" pumps available at this time are Medtronic system and the Tandem t-Slim. Both can work as a stand-alone pump, sensor-augmented pump, or hybrid closed loop system. Medtronic has its own sensor device—the Guardian connect. Tandem t-slim works with the DEXCOM CGM. The Omnipod system is a "tubeless" pump system available as a stand-alone pump and recently as a hybrid closed loop system (Figure 7.1).

3. Selecting a pump is a highly personalized choice. For most systems, insurers will only allow patients to change devices after the warranty on the current system has expired, which is typically 4.5 years. This makes it very important to choose wisely.

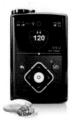 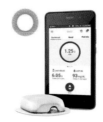 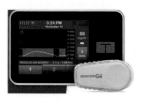

FIGURE 7.1. Comparison of Insulin Pumps. Image 1: Medtronic. Image 2: Omnipod. Image 3: DEXCOM.[7]

Websites such as "https://diabeteswise.org/#/" are helpful in that they present the systems in a balanced presentation and include feedback from existing users.

Return to the Case

Our patient was surprised to hear how much progress had been made on pump therapy for diabetes. He was very interested in a "tubeless" system but also wanted to be able to use a hybrid closed loop system. He went onto the Diabeteswise.org website and also checked out a couple of type 1 diabetes patient networks.

After doing sufficient research, he chose to start the Omnipod 5 system with the DEXCOM sensor. We submitted his paperwork. The DEXCOM was approved first, so he started this and received coverage for Omnipod about 1 month later. He has really enjoyed the system. He reports that it was hard at first to trust the system. But he has since discovered that he has smoother control and less hypoglycemia than he did with injections and SMBG. He is most impressed by how much less time he spends worrying about his diabetes.

Case Summary and Closing Points

People with type 1 diabetes can spend up to 5 hours/day on diabetes self-management.[9] Advanced technologies such as insulin pump therapy and hybrid closed loop systems help to reduce this burden by assisting in insulin dosing and improving safety. Moreover, research shows insulin pump therapy improves flexibility and quality of life for people with diabetes.[10] As exemplified by the DIY/Looping systems, the level of technology tools and assistant devices should only get better over time. While these technologies are not for everyone, they should at least be offered to all people with type 1 diabetes and those on complex basal and bolus insulin regimens.

References

1. Medtronic insulin pump home page. Accessed December 28, 2022. Medtronichttps://www.medtronic-diabetes.com/products/minimed-770g-insulin-pump-system.
2. Tandem insulin pump home page. Accessed December 28, 2022. https://www.tandemdiabetes.com/products/t-slim-x2-insulin-pump.
3. Omnipod insulin pump home page. Accessed December 28, 2022. Omnipodhttps://www.omnipod.com/.
4. DEXCOM glucose sensor home page. Accessed December 28, 2022. DEXCOMhttps://www.dexcom.com/.

5. Medtronic guardian sensor home page. Guardian connect. Accessed December 28, 2022. https://www.medtronicdiabetes.com/products/guardian-connect-continuous-glucose-monitoring-system.

6. *Diabeteswise.org.* Accessed December 28, 2022. https://diabeteswise.org/#/

7. Insulin pump devices-picture. Accessed December 28, 2022. https://www.google.com/search?q=comparison+of+insulin+pumps&rlz=1C5CHFA_enUS807US808&sxsrf=ALiCzsargMT7jv1Q_E8S3umLg1Rc_tf-og:1664203866543&source=lnms&tbm=isch&sa=X&ved=2ahUKEwiZ97HC2rL6AhWrElkFHebGCS4Q_AUoAXoECAIQAw&biw=1418&bih=669&dpr=2#imgrc=SXlXWmSYpYLeOM

8. DIY Looping System. Build your own closed loop system. Accessed December 28, 2022. https://diabetesstrong.com/diy-looping/

9. Shubrook JH, Brannan GD, Wapner A, Klein G, Schwartz FL. Time needed for diabetes self-care: nationwide survey of certified diabetes educators. *Diabetes Spectr.* 2018;31(3):267-271. doi:10.2337/ds17-0077

10. Abualula NA, Jacobsen KH, Milligan RA, Rodan MF, Conn VS. Evaluating diabetes educational interventions with a skill development component in adolescents with type 1 diabetes: a systematic review focusing on quality of life. *Diabetes Educ.* 2016;42(5):515-528. doi:10.1177/0145721716658356

Introduction

While we have tried to cover most of the common scenarios in diabetes care, there are still a few surprises. Here we discuss common but out-of-the-ordinary problems you may experience with your patients when providing diabetes care. Knowing to expect these will help you to be ready for the unexpected.

Case 1. Identifying Lipohypertrophy

"My insulin stopped working."

A 64-year-old man presents for a diabetes recheck. He has had diabetes for 12 years. He is not sure what is going on. His medications used to work well but lately; his fasting glucose has been climbing. His morning glucose readings are usually around 160 to 240 mg/dL. He does not check his glucose later in the day.

Med HX: type 2 diabetes, hypertension, dyslipidemia, degenerative joint disease in both knees, s/p bilateral knee replacement

Medications: metformin 1000 mg bid, insulin glargine 68 units per day, atorvastatin 40 mg daily, oral semaglutide 14 mg daily, valsartan/HCT 160/25 mg daily, diclofenac gel applied to each knee daily

Allergies: none

Family Medical History: family history (FH) of type 2 diabetes, hypertension (HTN)

Social History: lives with his spouse; retired janitor

Physical Exam: Ht. 5'7", Wt. 197 lb, BMI 30.9, P 66, R 15 BP 142/84

GEN: obese male with truncal obesity in no distress

HEENT: normal including thyroid exam

CV: normal

RESP: normal

Abdomen: soft nontender, large area of scar tissue noted to the left and the right of the umbilicus (lipohypertrophy) (Figure 8.1)

Extremities: normal peripheral pulses, bunions noted to both great toes, sensation to monofilament exam is diminished in both distal feet

Labs:

HbA1c: 8.9%

Random glucose: 244 mg/dL (1:30 PM)

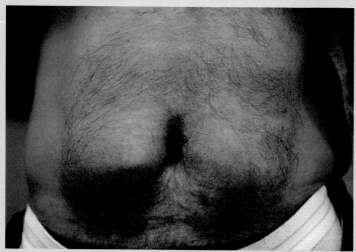

FIGURE 8.1. Image of lipohypertrophy. Mohammed SF, Kedir MS, Maru TT. (2015). Lipohypertrophy - The neglected area of concern in the much talked about diabetes. *Int J Diabetes Res.* 2015;4(2):38-42. doi:10.5923/j.diabetes.20150402.03.[1]

 CASE QUESTIONS

1. Is it possible that his insulin is not working?
2. What is causing his insulin not to work?
3. What cutaneous reactions can occur with repeated insulin injections?

ANSWERS AND EXPLANATIONS

1. Yes, of course. Most of these causes are preventable. There are several things that affect insulin absorption and efficacy. The first thing to do when you hear this complaint is to look at the injection sites (Figure 8.2). Be sure to palpate the injection sites as well.

    If the tissue is raised from scar tissue or there has been a loss of subcutaneous fat, this may affect insulin absorption. Further, people should only inject at sites that do not have scars (from previous surgery) or stretch marks, areas that do not have adequate subcutaneous fat, or areas that do not have enough vascular supply.

    If there are no obvious problems with the injection sites, the next step is to ask the patient to demonstrate taking an injection of insulin. The goal is to confirm the proper insulin injection technique. Potential problems include not inserting the needle deep enough, injecting it into an area without enough vascular flow, or not operating the syringe or insulin pen accurately.

    Finally, it is important to make sure that the insulin being used has not expired or denatured. We recommend that when a patient opens a pen or vial that they

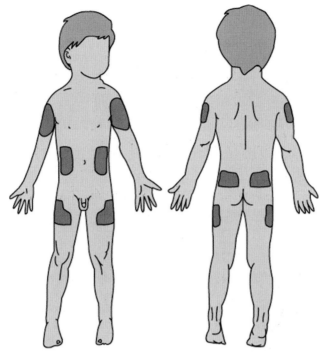

FIGURE 8.2. Potential injection sites. (Used with permission from Silbert-Flagg J. *Maternal & Child Health Nursing.* 9th ed. Wolters Kluwer; 2022.)[2]

write the date opened on it with a sharpie. Most insulins are ok to use for 28 days after opening. While pens do not have to be refrigerated, it is important that the insulin not be exposed to extremes of temperature as this can denature or inactivate the insulin.

2. In this patient's case, he has been injecting into the same spot for a long time and has, as a result, built up scar tissue. The term for this is lipohypertrophy. This scar tissue does not allow normal absorption of the injected insulin. Some people experience no noticeable insulin effects, while others will experience irregular absorption of insulin.

   Best practices for people who have lipohypertrophy are to avoid this area for at least 3 months to allow for possible normalization of tissue.

3. With proper injection techniques, these reactions can be largely prevented. However, you can see either a build-up of scar tissue (lipohypertrophy) (Figures 8.3 and 8.4A and B) or a breakdown of the subcutaneous fat (lipoatrophy)[4] (Figure 8.5).

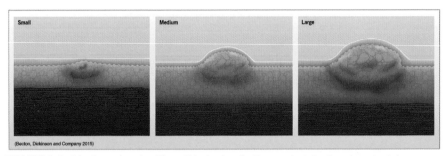

FIGURE 8.3. Lipohypertrophy. Venn-Wycherley A. Suspect, detect and protect: lessons from a lipohypertrophy workshop for children's nurses. *Nurs Child Young People.* 2015;27(9):21-5. doi:10.7748/ncyp.27.9.21.s23.[3]

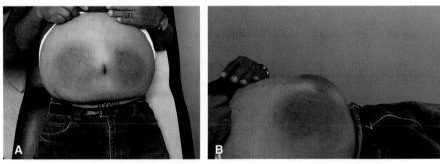

FIGURE 8.4. A and B, Insulin-medicated lipohypertrophy. A, Front view of Lipohypertrophy. B, Side view of Lipohypertrophy—you can see how area is raised.

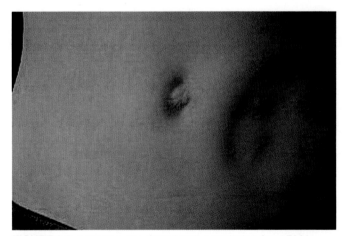

FIGURE 8.5. Lipoatrophy. (Used with permission from BMJ Publishing Group Ltd.)[4]

Case Summary and Closing Points

Improper insulin administration can affect a person's glucose control. It is important to show your patients where they can safely inject their insulin and that they must rotate or move sites regularly. When patients are injecting (insulin or other medications) they should avoid scar tissue, stretch marks, areas with little subcutaneous fat, and areas of low vascularity. Correct insulin techniques help patients receive the optimal and expected benefits from the medicine they are administering.

References

1. Injection sites. https://mysteadyshot.com/pages/injection-sites (different -ok to use other version
2. Lipohypertrophy case.
3. Lipohypertrophy cartoon.
4. Babiker A, Datta V. Lipoatrophy with insulin analogues in type I diabetes. *Arch Dis Child.* 2011;96:101-102.

Case 2.	Glucose Testing and Diabetes Supply Snafus

"My friends say I have an A1c machine for home."

A 48-year-old British man presents for a diabetes recheck. He has had diabetes for 8 years. He recently returned from a trip to England. Now, he reports that something is not "right" with his glucometer. Typically, he has been able to meet glucose goals. He knew that he would run higher during his vacation as he planned to enjoy all his favorite foods and beers. So, he took the precaution of visiting a local doctor during the visit. Since then, his readings have not made sense. He has been getting readings of 4.8 to 10.0.

When he returned to the United States, he showed his friend the meter he received from the English clinician. The friend said that the doctor had given him "one of those home A1c machines," which he thought explained the low readings. The patient does not think the meter has been altered and is seeking confirmation.

Med HX: type 2 diabetes, hypertension, dyslipidemia, depression

Medications: metformin 1000 mg bid, pioglitazone 30 mg daily, acarbose 50 mg tid qac, atorvastatin 40 mg daily, ramipril 5 mg daily

Allergies: none

Family Medical History: FH of type 2 diabetes, HTN, Alzheimer disease in mom

Social History: lives alone, author

Physical Exam: Ht. 5′9″, Wt. 193 lb, BMI 28.5, P 85, R 19, BP 136/80

GEN: obese male with truncal obesity in no distress

HEENT: normal including thyroid exam

CV: normal

RESP: normal

Abdomen: soft nontender, no masses

Extremities: normal peripheral pulses, normal sensation to monofilament exam to both distal feet

Labs:

Current A1c: 8.4%, last HbA1c 6 months ago was 7.1%.

Patient's meter reading: 10.0

Office glucose reading: 180

CASE QUESTIONS

1. What is the issue with his glucometer?
2. What are other common problems with glucometers?
3. What are common problems people have with supplies?

ANSWERS AND EXPLANATIONS

1. The first thing to do is to examine the meter settings. Upon review, we discovered that the glucose units had been changed from mg/dL (US) to mmol/L (as used by most of the rest of the world). Since most people in the United States use imperial (or mass concentration) units, the metric (or molar) units for glucose will likely appear foreign. The good news is that it is easy to change the settings. Further, there is a simple conversion for switching between these units.

   To get mg/dL (US) from mmol/L, multiply by 18. Conversely, to switch from mg/dL to mmol/L, divide by 18.

   Our patient had a 10.0 mmol/L reading. We multiply the reading by 18 and determine that his US-based reading is 180 mg/dL.

2. Most people can work a glucometer without difficulty, yet some problems do arise. These include failing to change the settings with time changes that occur at daylight savings time. Most meters need to be set to the correct time and date or the data from the meters cannot be downloaded.

   Another problem arises when users fail to test the meter with the control solution. All commercially approved meters must meet national standards for accuracy. However, there are some actions that can make the meter reading less accurate. All meters should be tested with a control solution with each new container of test strips. The control solution should also be refilled 90 days after opening. If the control solution is not used to calibrate the meter, the readings can drift.

   Inaccurate readings can occur when users do not use clean hands when handling their meter. The correct technique is to clean and dry the testing site before performing glucose testing. A reading can be dramatically affected if obtained with unwashed hands.

   Failing to use different sites for glucose checks can be problematic. If a person only uses one site for glucose monitoring, the skin can become callused and thickened (as discussed earlier), which may make it harder to test in that area in the future. Asking the patient to switch to new glucose monitoring sites will resolve this.

Finally, some people use an inadequate setting on the lancing device to get enough blood to test. When we are helping a patient with a new setup on a glucose measuring device, we explicitly show them how to adjust the lancing device depth. We usually advise patients to start with the middle setting and then show them how to adjust for comfort and efficacy.

3. One of the most common problems experienced by people with diabetes is not being able to get needed supplies. This is usually because the prescription was not written correctly, or the prescription did not have an ICD code attached. These and other common problems (and solutions) are listed in the following text.

Glucose Testing Supplies

When you write for these supplies, be sure to include, at a minimum, the lancets and glucose test strips. Ideally you are also writing for alcohol swabs to clean fingers. The number of each supply should match the number of glucose tests you are prescribing per day. Most of these supplies come in multiples of 25 or 50. Be sure to include a diagnosis code that supports the use of this equipment.

I write all testing supplies for 1 year. This allows the patient to have the supplies they need and reduces the number of random calls and requests for refills.

Sample RX

1. XX Brand Glucose test strips. #200. (3-month supply) Sig. fingerstick glucose 2 times per day. ICD code: E11.65, E16.2. 3 refills
2. XX Brand Lancets. #100. (3-month supply) Sig. fingerstick glucose 2 times per day. ICD code: E11.65, E16.2. 3 refills
3. Alcohol swabs #200. (3-month supply) Sig. fingerstick glucose 2 times per day. ICD code: E11.65, E16.2. 3 refills

Insulin Prescribing Problems

There are two common problems with insulin prescriptions. The first is not providing the needed tools to deliver insulin. If you are writing for insulin vials, you must also write for insulin syringes. Syringes come in three different volumes: 0.3 mL (holds up to 30 units), 0.5 mL (holds up to 50 units), and 1 mL (holds up to 100 units). It is important to make sure you provide a syringe that can hold the amount of insulin the person is supposed to inject. Otherwise, the person will need to take multiple injections for a single dose of insulin. The second issue is specifying what length needle you want on the syringe. To make things simple, I always use the shortest needles available on the insulin syringe and insulin pens. This is usually 5/32″ or 0.4 mm.

Sample RX

Insulin syringes 0.5 mL, #100 (1-month supply). Inject 35 units tid qac. E10.65, I10.

Additional problems include not writing for enough insulin for the given prescription or not providing the maximum daily dose if the insulin dose varies. It is important to write for the correct volume of insulin to match what the patient will be taking. Otherwise, they may run out of insulin early. This can result in gaps in medication, extra co-pays, and more trips to the pharmacy. To provide the correct volume of insulin, take the daily dose and multiply this by 30 or 90 days depending on the length of the prescription. Notice that we have included the ICD code as well in the prescriptions below.

Example: The patient is taking 50 units daily of insulin glargine by pen and insulin aspart 15 units per meal tid by pen. We want to provide him with a 3-month supply (90 days).

50 units/day × 90 days = 4500 units glargine.

*You can write the quantity as units or you can convert it into volume. **Pro-tip:** Each pen holds 300 units, Therefore: 4500 units/300 units/pen = 15 pens.*

For his mealtime insulin, he takes 15 units per meal. That is 45 units per day.

45 units/day × 90 days = 4050 units. Each pen has 300 units.

4050 units/300 units/pen = 13.5 pens. As you probably know we cannot prescribe ½ a pen. Pro-tip: Most insulin pens come in boxes of 5 so we will end up writing for 15 pens again.

The Prescription Would Look Like This

Insulin glargine U100. Dispense 45 pens (90 day supply). Take 50 units once daily in the evening. E11.65.

Insulin aspart. Dispense 45 pens (90 day supply). Take 15 units before each meal tid. E11.65.

Pen needles. Dispense: #400 (90 day supply). Inject insulin 4 times per day. E11.65.

One Last Insulin Issue

Many people who take mealtime insulin also take correction as part of their mealtime dose. This means that the dose may vary significantly from day to day. The pharmacy will share the directions for correction dosing, but the prescription must have a maximum daily dose to ensure an adequate supply. If the max daily dose is not on the prescription, the pharmacist will not know how much to dispense, and the prescription will be returned to the prescriber.

Let's modify the prescription above for insulin aspart. This patient takes 15 units before each meal but also takes a correction dose if his glucose is high. The correction scale recommends to add 2 extra units for every 50 mg/dL the reading is above 150 mg/dL.

The Prescription Would Look Like This

Insulin aspart. Dispense 30 pens (90-day supply). Take 15 units before each meal tid plus 2 units for every 50 above 150. Max daily dose 90 units/day. E11.65.

Pen needles: 4 mm (nano) Dispense: #400 (90-day supply). Inject insulin 4 times per day. E11.65.

This may seem rather complicated the first few times you write these prescriptions. You will find, though, that the process does get easier with repetition and will eventually become second nature. Writing prescriptions well means fewer phone calls from the pharmacy.

Below are suggestions to make the calculation for insulin doses easier:

- **Pro-tips:**
  1. When writing for insulin pens, every 45 units taken daily requires 1 box of 5 pens per month.
  2. For people who take insulin by vial, every 30 units taken daily requires 1 vial per month.
  3. Write all testing supplies for 1 year. If done correctly, refills will be easy year after year.

Case Summary and Closing Points

The person with diabetes will need supplies to test their glucose and to take their insulin. These must be prescribed correctly to ensure uninterrupted access to those items needed for self-care. These simple steps can make all the difference in the world for your patients.

Case 3. Make a Sick Day Plan

"I do not know why I am running high."

A 66-year-old man presents for an acute visit. He reports that normally his diabetes is well controlled, but he got gastroenteritis 2 days ago and he has been having nausea, vomiting, and diarrhea ever since. He was not eating and did not want to take his medications. He has been running very high and he is not sure what he should do. He has had diverticulitis before, and this can make him sick for about a week, but this is worse than that.

Normally his AM readings are 120 to 150 mg/dL and random glucose readings are 100 to 160 mg/dL. This week he has not been below 160 mg/dL and he is not eating.

Med HX: type 2 diabetes, hypertension, gastroesophageal reflux disease, dyslipidemia, chronic obstructive pulmonary disease (COPD), diverticulitis

Medications: metformin 1000 mg bid, glipizide 5 mg bid, canagliflozin 300 mg daily, simvastatin 40 mg daily, combivent 2 puff bid, amlodipine 5 mg daily, chlorthalidone 25 mg daily, omeprazole 40 mg daily

Allergies: none

Family Medical History: diabetes and COPD runs in family

Social History: lives with his spouse

Physical Exam: Ht. 5′6″, Wt. 161 lb, BMI 26, P 80, R 22, BP 106/74

GEN: alert male in mild distress and appears uncomfortable and dehydrated

HEENT: normal including thyroid exam

CV: normal

RESP: prolongation of expiration

Abdomen: soft, mild diffuse tenderness

Extremities: normal peripheral pulses, no skin changes, sensation to monofilament is normal

Psych: affect and mood normal

Labs: last HbA1c—7.2%

Current glucose: 188 mg/dL

 CASE QUESTIONS

1. Can this illness make his glucose run higher?
2. What should he do with his medications?
3. How do you devise a "sick day plan" for when this happens again?

 ANSWERS AND EXPLANATIONS

1. Any illness or significant stressor can make glucose run higher. The tendency is more pronounced when the illness is systemic. In fact, many patients with diabetes find that the change in glucose can be an early warning of some other illness (like gout for example). In this case, his gastrointestinal illness is a stressor to the body and in response, the body mobilizes its glucose stores in a fight or flight response.

    Many patients are confused when they know that they have not eaten but their glucose is still high. Further, many patients are afraid to take diabetes medications if they are not eating. Reflexively, patients will skip medications for fear of dropping too low.

2. It is important to develop a plan for your patients who have multiple comorbidities and are at risk for exacerbations or hospitalization. Often, we will instruct patients to skip certain medications that can have more risk when the person is acutely ill. For example, this patient takes metformin. This medication is often stopped when people are hospitalized due to the risk of acute kidney injury. His use of glipizide will depend on what his glucose is doing. If he is running higher, he may need to continue this. However, if he is unable to eat, he may need to hold this due to the risk of hypoglycemia. We recommend that patients seek medical

advice under these circumstances to determine the safest way to proceed during this acute illness.

3. Most patients with diabetes should have a "sick day plan."[1] The plan should outline how to manage diabetes when sick or unable to eat or drink. This is important as the dosing of medication can be complicated especially when associated with hypoglycemia.[2]

Here are our recommendations for diabetes sick days:

1. Check glucose more often—if you are running higher than normal or dropping low, you may need to adjust your medication. Consult your healthcare professional for advice.
2. Stay hydrated—good hydration helps distribute medication and limits potential acute kidney damage.
3. If you are unclear as to whether you should take your medication, please call the office or the doctor on call for clarification.

Some general rules regarding oral medications:

1. If you are having severe nausea, vomiting or diarrhea, hold off from taking metformin.
2. Sulfonylureas should only be continued if glucose remains high despite decreased oral intake.
3. Sodium-glucose cotransporter-2 (SGLT-2) inhibitors may need to be temporarily stopped in an acute illness as they can contribute to worsening dehydration when the person is hyperglycemic and in rare cases lead to euglycemic diabetic ketoacidosis (DKA).
4. Insulin is often the safest medication to use when acutely ill.

Resources for Sick Day Guidelines

1. ADA: Accessed December 30, 2022. https://diabetes.org/diabetes/treatment-care/planning-sick-days[1]
2. CDC: Accessed December 30, 2022. https://www.cdc.gov/diabetes/managing/flu-sick-days.html#:~:text=Follow%20these%20additional%20steps%20when,eat%20as%20you%20normally%20would[2]
3. ADCES—Sick day type 1 PDF. Accessed December 30, 2022. https://www.diabeteseducator.org/docs/default-source/education-and-career/sickday_adult.pdf?sfvrsn=2[3]
4. Nebraska Med—Sick day type 2 PDF[4]

Case Summary and Closing Points

People with diabetes are susceptible to changes in glucose when they get sick with an acute illness. Each person may respond slightly differently, so it is important to discuss the scenario with your patients and develop sick day plans. The sick day plan should provide guidance for glucose monitoring, hydration, and any medication changes that are needed.

References

1. American Diabetes Association Planning for Sick Days. Available at: https://diabetes.org/diabetes/treatment-care/planning-sick-days
2. Centers for Disease Control and Prevention Managing Diabetes on Sick Days. Available at: https://www.cdc.gov/diabetes/managing/flu-sick-days.html
3. American Association of Diabetes Care and Education Specialists: Sick day type 1 diabetes. Available at: https://www.diabeteseducator.org/docs/default-source/education-and-career/sickday_adult.pdf?s-fvrsn=2
4. Nebraska Med- Sick day management for type 2 diabetes PDF. Available at: https://www.nebraskamed.com/sites/default/files/documents/Diabetes/9212_Sick_Day_Type%202.pdf

---

Case 4.   Steroid-Associated Hyperglycemia

"My asthma flared up again."

A 26-year-old man presents to establish care. He has had type 1 diabetes since the age of 18 years. He reports that most of the time he has a good handle on his diabetes. He was admitted for DKA when he was diagnosed but he has not had any hospitalizations (for hyperglycemia or hypoglycemia) for his diabetes since.

The only time when it gets really hard to manage his diabetes, he explains, is when his asthma flares up. His readings start to climb early in an asthma attack but when he needs to take steroids, his sugars really climb. He as though he is chasing the high readings without effect.

Med HX: type 1 diabetes, moderate persistent asthma

Medications: insulin degludec 27 units daily, insulin glulisine 1:9 carb ratio breakfast, 1:10 carb ratio for lunch, dinner and snacks. Correction 1 unit for every 20 mg/dL about 120 mg/dL. Symbicort 80/4.5 1 to 2 puffs bid and q4h prn.

Allergies: none

Family Medical History: parents are healthy, no sibs

Social History: lives with his two friends, both knowledgeable about diabetes; works as a librarian

Physical Exam: Ht. 5′9″, Wt. 161 lb, BMI 23.8, P 66, R 14, BP 106/74

GEN: alert male in no distress

HEENT: normal including thyroid exam

CV: normal

RESP: normal

Abdomen: soft nontender, injection sites with no lipohypertrophy

Extremities: normal peripheral pulses, normal sensation to monofilament exam to both distal feet

Psych: affect and mood normal

CASE QUESTIONS

1. Can his asthma make his glucose run higher?
2. How should you treat steroid-associated hyperglycemia?
3. How do you decrease the insulin as they get better?

 ## ANSWERS AND EXPLANATIONS

1. As established in the previous case studies, many things, other than food and insulin, affect glucose levels. In fact, many people with diabetes discover that their glucose levels can serve as an early warning system when other illnesses start. While this is nonspecific, it is a sign that the body is under stress and trying to mobilize glucose to handle the source of the stress.

2. This patient is on chronic use of inhaled corticosteroids. It is strongly recommended that these inhalers be used as directed. Further, users of these inhalers should rinse their mouths out thoroughly after use to reduce systemic absorption of corticosteroids. Even with these precautions, though, some people can see mild glucose-raising effects from steroid inhalers.

   When this patient has exacerbations of his asthma, he sometimes needs oral corticosteroids. While these are necessary to address his asthma, they significantly raise his glucose. For people with type 1 diabetes, this can be especially challenging as it can sometimes trigger a DKA episode.

   Helping this patient means developing a plan to address steroid-associated hyperglycemia. While studies are limited to advising treatment, the following are strategies that can help people in this situation and should be considered when devising a plan.

   People on oral therapies only (type 2 diabetes) may need to take insulin temporarily. Often, oral therapies cannot cover significant hyperglycemia. For prednisone, NPH insulin is often used as it peaks about the same time the effect of prednisone peaks. The dose can start at 0.1 units/mg dose of prednisone and is dosed at the same time as each prednisone dose.[1]

   It is not uncommon for people on insulin to need to increase their insulin dose when they are started on corticosteroids. The largest increases are needed for mealtime and correction dosing only. Many people may need to double the amount of correction insulin they are taking with their meals and for correction. If the steroid regimen is prolonged more than 3 to 5 days, basal insulin may also need to be increased.

3. There is no simple answer to this challenging question. This will depend on several factors including the type of diabetes the patient has, how sensitive they are to insulin, the length and the dose of the corticosteroid, and the duration of the illness. Many people will try to reduce the insulin dose as the corticosteroid is being tapered and most people will stop the elevated dose of insulin once the corticosteroid is stopped.

Case Summary and Closing Points

Corticosteroids are important medications for several illnesses, but they are also associated with widespread side effects. In people with diabetes who take corticosteroids, significant and prolonged hyperglycemia can be seen. Consequently, it is important to develop a plan with patients to address steroid-associated hyperglycemia.

References

1. Elena C, Chiara M, Angelica B, et al. Hyperglycemia and diabetes induced by glucocorticoids in nondiabetic and diabetic patients: revision of literature and personal considerations. *Curr Pharm Biotechnol.* 2018;19(15):1210-1220.

Case 5.   Diabetes Complications—Microvascular—Retinopathy, Nephropathy, Neuropathy

A 40-year-old woman presents for a diabetes recheck. She was diagnosed with diabetes 6 months ago. She is doing everything she can to prevent problems. Her family has had a difficult history with diabetes. Both her mom and maternal aunt died from diabetes complications, and she does not want diabetes to take her.

Med HX: type 2 diabetes, hypertension, dyslipidemia

Medications: metformin 1000 mg bid, dapagliflozin 10 mg daily, rosuvastatin 20 mg daily

Allergies: none

Family Medical History: FH of type 2 diabetes, premature heart disease in dad and brother

Social History: lives with his spouse, retired janitor

Physical Exam: Ht. 5'5", Wt. 162 lb, BMI 27, P 88, R 16 BP 112/68

GEN: obese male with truncal obesity in no distress

HEENT: normal including thyroid exam

CV: normal

RESP: normal

Abdomen: soft nontender, no masses

Extremities: normal peripheral pulses, normal sensation to monofilament exam in both distal feet

Labs:

HbA1c: 6.8%

Random glucose: 128 mg/dL (10:40 AM)

CASE QUESTIONS

1. What are the most common complications associated with diabetes?
2. What are the recommended screening tests for these complications?
3. What are the core concepts regarding complication prevention?

 ANSWERS AND EXPLANATIONS

1. Diabetes is a leading cause of microvascular complications. These include retinopathy (the leading cause of legal blindness), nephropathy (the leading cause of end-stage renal disease resulting in dialysis), and neuropathy (the leading cause of nontraumatic amputations).[1,2]

   While these are the most common complications, the leading cause of death for people with diabetes is cardiovascular disease. People with diabetes have a two- to fourfold higher risk of cardiovascular disease.[3]

   For all these complications, it is most important to know that there are no classic "early symptoms" to let people know that they are at risk. Therefore, it is essential to do evidence-based screening tests to identify early signs of these complications.

2. All people with type 2 diabetes should be screened for microvascular complications starting at diagnosis.

Retinopathy[1]

Screening for diabetes-related retinopathy should start at diagnosis for people with type 2 diabetes and by 5 years after diagnosis in people with type 1 diabetes.

Diabetes-retinopathy should include a dilated eye exam completed annually by an eye specialist. Retinal photography can be used as well to improve access to retinopathy screening. If used, timely referral to an eye specialist is critical.

If a person with stable glucose control has two or more consecutive normal readings, then the diabetes-related retinopathy screening can be moved to every 1 to 2 years as long as it continues to stay normal.

Pregnancy is a high-risk time for women with diabetes. If possible, an eye exam should be completed before the woman becomes pregnant, during the first trimester, and then monitored every trimester and at least 1 year postpartum.

Nephropathy (Diabetes-Related Kidney Disease)

Screening for diabetes-related nephropathy should start at diagnosis for people with type 2 diabetes and by 5 years after diagnosis in people with type 1 diabetes.

Screening for diabetes-related kidney disease should include **BOTH** an annual assessment of estimated glomerular filtration rate (eGFR) and urinary excretion of albumin (UACr). This is obtained from a blood test and specific urine analysis.

These screening tests should occur annually and unless one of the tests becomes abnormal: then the screening should be completed at least twice annually to guide treatment therapy.

				Persistent albuminuria categories Description and range		
				A1	A2	A3
				Normal to mildly increased	Moderately increased	Severely increased
				<30 mg/g <3 mg/mmol	30–300 mg/g 3–30 mg/mmol	>300 mg/g >30 mg/mmol
GFR categories (ml/min/ 1.73 m²) Description and range	G1	Normal or high	≥90		Monitor	Refer*
	G2	Mildly decreased	60–89		Monitor	Refer*
	G3a	Mildly to moderately decreased	45–59	Monitor	Monitor	Refer
	G3b	Moderately to severely decreased	30–44	Monitor	Monitor	Refer
	G4	Severely decreased	15–29	Refer*	Refer*	Refer
	G5	Kidney failure	<15	Refer	Refer	Refer

FIGURE 8.6. The KDIGO heat map for chronic kidney disease. (Used with permission from Kidney Disease Improving Global Outcomes (KDIGO).)

If the patient develops diabetes-related chronic kidney disease, it is important to stage this condition using the recommendations from the KDIGO guidelines. The staging includes both an eGFR stage and an albuminuria stage as represented in the KDIGO heat map[4] (Figure 8.6).

Neuropathy[1]

The American Diabetes Association recommends that for people with type 1 diabetes, these screenings should begin 5 years after initial diagnosis. If there is evidence of loss of protective sensation in a visual inspection of the feet should occur at every visit.

There are multiple forms of diabetes-related neuropathy. Symmetric sensory poly-neuropathy is the most common form. Up to 50% of people who have peripheral neuropathy may be asymptomatic proving the need for screening.

Diabetes-related peripheral neuropathy can present as unpleasant sensations in the feet including pain, burning, and tingling or can present as numbness and loss of protective sensation. Because of the different presentations, it is important to test each of the fiber types to identify these problems.

Neuropathy screening for neuropathy should include an annual foot exam that includes inspection of both lower legs and feet looking for skin changes, sores, calluses, or ulcerations; assessment of either temperature or print prick sensation (small fibers assessment); vibration sensation using a 120 Hz tuning fork (large fiber assessment); a vascular exam; and checking for sensory loss with the use of a 10-g monofilament exam.

3. **Retinopathy**[1]
The cornerstones of diabetes-related retinopathy treatment include glucose control, blood pressure control, and if needed pan-retinal laser photocoagulation or intravitreal injections of anti–vascular endothelial growth factor agents.

It is important to let your patients know that these treatments for diabetes-related retinopathy are vision sparing but they do not improve the vision acutely.

Nephropathy[2]
The cornerstones of diabetes-related kidney disease treatment include glucose control, blood pressure control, weight loss, moderation of protein intake with a preference for plant-based protein, and early referral to nephrology. Referral to nephrology is recommended for all patients who have chronic kidney disease stage 3B or albuminuria stage A3.

For patients who have hypertension or evidence of albuminuria, the initiation of an angiotensin-converting enzyme inhibitor or angiotensin receptor blocker (not both) should be started and titrated to the max tolerated dose.

To address residual risk for progression of diabetes-related kidney disease and cardiovascular disease, agents with proven benefits to reduce these risks should be considered in these patients. These include SGLT-2 inhibitors, glucagon-like peptide (GLP)-1 receptor agonists, and mineral corticoid receptor antagonists.

Neuropathy[1]
The cornerstones of treating diabetes-related peripheral neuropathy include glucose control, smoking cessation, symptom control with pharmacotherapy, and protection of the foot and skin with well-fit shoes or custom-made orthotics.

Case Summary and Closing Points

While much of the work for diabetes is day-to-day glucose management, the goal of this work is to prevent long-term microvascular and macrovascular complications. These complications are typically silent at first and the only way to find them early is to follow the recommended screening protocols. This will allow for early identification and treatment.

References

1. American Diabetes Association 2002 Standards of Care for People with Diabetes. Chapter 12: Retinopathy, Neuropathy and Foot care. Available at: https://diabetesjournals.org/care/article/45/Supplement_1/S185/138917/12-Retinopathy-Neuropathy-and-Foot-Care-Standards
2. American Diabetes Association 2002 Standards of Care for People with Diabetes. Chapter 11: Chronic Kidney Disease and Risk Management. Available at: https://diabetesjournals.org/care/article/45/Supplement_1/S175/138914/11-Chronic-Kidney-Disease-and-Risk-Management
3. American Diabetes Association 2002 Standards of Care for People with Diabetes. Chapter 10: Cardiovascular Disease and Risk Management. Available at: https://diabetesjournals.org/care/article/45/Supplement_1/S144/138910/10-Cardiovascular-Disease-and-Risk-Management
4. KDIGO 2022 Clinical Practice Guideline for diabetes management in chronic kidney disease. Available at: https://kdigo.org/wp-content/uploads/2022/03/KDIGO-2022-Diabetes-Management-GL_Public-Review-draft_1Mar2022.pdf

Case 6. Nonalcoholic Fatty Liver Disease

"Is it safe for me to take a statin?"

A 61-year-old woman presents for a diabetes recheck. She has had diabetes for 12 years. She reports that she tries to keep up with her diabetes but finds it to be a lot of work. She was recently seen in the emergency room for belly pain which, she says, turned out to be gas pain. The ER doctor told her that she has a "fatty liver," that some of her tests were elevated, and that she should talk to her diabetes doctor about cholesterol medicine.

Med HX: type 2 diabetes, hypertension, dyslipidemia, osteoarthritis both thumbs, frequent urinary tract infections

Medications: metformin 1000 mg bid, insulin glargine 30 units per day, atorvastatin 20 mg daily, cranberry capsules prn, amlodipine 5 mg daily

Allergies: none

Family Medical History: FH of type 2 diabetes, HTN, sister has cirrhosis (but never drank alcohol)

Social History: lives with her spouse

Physical Exam: Ht. 5'5", Wt. 202 lb, BMI 33.6, P 84, R 20, BP 106/70

GEN: obese female with truncal obesity in no distress

HEENT: normal including thyroid exam

CV: normal

RESP: normal

Abdomen: soft, mild RUQ and epigastric tenderness on deep palpation

Extremities: normal peripheral pulses, calluses noted on the later aspects of both feet, sensation intact to monofilament exam

Labs:

Lipid Panel	Value	Reference Range
Cholesterol, total	248	125-200 mg/dL
Triglycerides	256	<150 mg/dL
LDL (calculated)	108	<130 mg/dL
HDL cholesterol	30	>40 mg/dL men; > 50 mg/dL women
Non-HDL cholesterol	158	<130 mg/dL

Other Labs	Value	Reference Range
HbA1c	6.4%	<5.7% (normal)
Urine albumin/creatinine ratio (UACr)	20 mg/g	<30 mg/g

Comprehensive Metabolic Panel	Value	Reference Range
Sodium	138	136-145 mmol/L
Potassium, serum	4.1	3.5-5.3 mmol/L
Chloride, serum	104	98-110 mmol/L
Carbon dioxide (CO_2)	24	19-30 mmol/L
Urea nitrogen, blood (BUN)	21	7-25 mg/dL
Creatinine, serum	1.2	0.5-1.10 mg/dL
eGFR	88	>60 mL/min/1.73 m^2
Glucose, serum	104	65-99 mg/dL
Calcium, serum	9.0	8.6-10.2 mg/dL
Protein, total	7.1	6.1-8.1 g/dL
Albumin	4.3	3.6-4.1 g/dL
Globulin	2.8	1.9-3.7 g/dL
AST (SGOT)	48	10-35 U/L
ALT (SGPT)	52	6-29 U/L
Bilirubin, total	0.7	0.2-1.2 mg/dL
Alkaline phosphatase	100	33-115 U/L

CBC	Value	Reference Range
White blood cell count	8.0	3.8-10.8 thousand/µL
Red blood cell count	4.8	3.8-5.10 million/µL
Hemoglobin	14.3	12.6-17 g/dL
Hematocrit	48%	37%-51%
MCV	91	80-100 fL
MCH	29.9	27-33 pg
MCHC	32.9	32-36 g/dL
RDW	12.7	1%-15%
Platelet count	167	140-400 thousand/µL

Ⓠ CASE QUESTIONS

1. What is the recommended evaluation for her "fatty liver" and elevated transaminases?
2. What are the guidelines for screening for NAFLD/NASH?
3. What is the recommendation regarding diagnosis and referral?
4. What are the recommended treatments for this patient?

ANSWERS AND EXPLANATIONS

1. It is important to recognize that fat infiltration in the viscera is not normal and not diagnostic. There are several causes. If possible, the cause should be identified. Nonalcoholic fatty liver disease (NAFLD) is a common disorder affecting 28% of the general population and more than 60% of people with diabetes. It might be better named a cardiometabolic liver disease. NAFLD is a spectrum of disorders characterized by excessive fat infiltration in the liver in the absence of other known liver disorders. It has two components, NAFL—the presence of >5% fat in the liver without evidence of inflammation, fibrosis, or cirrhosis and nonalcoholic steatohepatitis (NASH)—which is present when inflammation is evident and can include progressive bridging fibrosis and cirrhosis.

    The name NAFLD comes from a time when the condition was present in people who reported that they did not consume alcohol but has histologic findings that were identical to alcoholic liver disease.

    For many years this condition was identified with a diagnosis of exclusion. The diagnosis could only be made by liver biopsy. With the number of people affected by this condition, a less invasive and more cost-effective algorithm was desperately needed.

2. The American Gastroenterology Association in conjunction with the American College of Osteopathic Family Physicians, American Academy of Family Physicians, American Association of Clinical Endocrinologists, American Association for the Study of Liver Diseases, American Diabetes Association, The Endocrine Society, and The Obesity Society recommend that all adults with type 2 diabetes be screened for NAFLD.[1]

    They also recommend that adults with two or more risk factors of metabolic syndrome also be screened. Finally, they recommend that people who find out that they have fatty liver on imaging or those with elevated transaminases also undergo screening.[1] These patients should have a routine history and physical for advanced liver disease.

    The recommended first step in screening is the use of a noninvasive test called the Fib-4 calculation. This can be completed with a patient's age, ALT, AST, and platelet levels. The Fib-4 score is divided into low risk, high risk, and indeterminate risk categories.[2] The risk stratification helps to determine the next step in the algorithm.

    Our patient has a Fib-4 score of 2.43, which is in the indeterminate range but on the higher end of this category (Figure 8.7).

3. For patients with elevated transaminases, it is important to rule out other causes of liver disease such as excessive alcohol intake, viral hepatitis, and autoimmune liver disease.

    If these are not present, move to the next step of the evaluation. For those with low-risk Fib-4 (low risk to advance to liver fibrosis and cirrhosis), it is recommended that the patient is screened again every 2 to 3 years.

    For those with indeterminate and high-risk Fib-4 scores, the next step is to evaluate for liver stiffness. This cannot be done with an ultrasound alone but

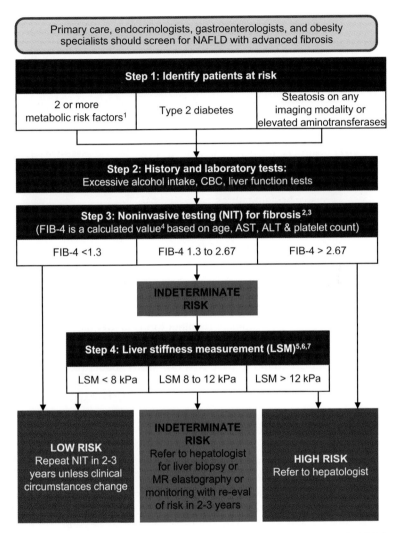

FIGURE 8.7. Screening for advanced fibrosis related to NAFLD/NASH.[2]

requires specialized elastography, which measures liver stiffness. This is also non-invasive and can be done at a local hospital or with a hepatologist. See Figure 8.7 for the risk scoring for the Fibroscan (liver stiffness measurement [LSM]). Our patient had an LSM of 12.8 kPa, which puts her in the highest risk category. Thus, she should be referred to a hepatologist for liver-directed treatment (Figure 8.8). The Enhanced Liver Fibrosis test has become avialable in the US and may be an alternative to the Fibroscan for determining risk in those with indeterminate risk of advanced NASH.[3]

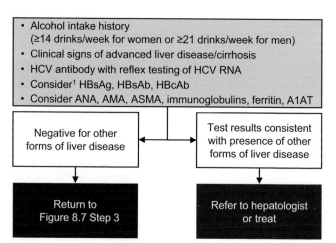

Footnote: **1.** Not everyone should be tested for Hep B core antibodies due to high positivity but uncertain clinical significance.

Abbreviations: **HBsAg** = hepatitis B surface antigen, **HBsAb** = hepatitis B surface antibody, **HBcAb** = hepatitis B core antibody, **HCV** = hepatitis C virus, **ANA** = antinuclear antibodies, **AMA** = antimitochondrial antibodies, **ASMA** = anti-smooth muscle antibodies, **A1AT** = alpha-1 antitrypsin

FIGURE 8.8. Evaluate for other forms of liver disease.[2]

4. All patients who are found to have NAFLD/NASH should receive education on therapeutic lifestyle change with the primary goal of weight loss and cardiovascular risk reduction. The limitation or cessation of alcohol consumption should also be reinforced.

While much of the concern about NAFLD/NASH centers around liver-specific complications, the number one cause of death among these patients is cardiovascular disease. Weight loss has been shown to have substantial benefits for these patients including a reduction in progression to advanced liver disease and, in some cases, reversal of early fibrosis. Cardiovascular risk reduction can include improved glucose and blood pressure control. Further, it has been shown that statins are beneficial for these patients and should not be withheld in people with mild elevations of transaminases.

All people with NAFLD should be treated by a team that includes the primary care clinician, dietitian, and other specialists based upon the patient's comorbidities. People with type 2 diabetes and NAFLD should have specific diabetes pharmacotherapy that has been shown to treat diabetes and provide benefits for people with NAFLD. These treatments include pioglitazone and the GLP-1RA (Figure 8.9).

	LOW RISK FIB-4 < 1.3 or LSM < 8 kPa or liver biopsy F0-F1	INDETERMINATE RISK FIB-4 1.3 - 2.67 and/or LSM 8 - 12 kPa and liver biopsy not available	HIGH RISK[1] FIB-4 > 2.67 or LSM > 12 kPa or liver biopsy F2-F4
	Management by PCP, dietician, endocrinologist, cardiologist, others	Management by hepatologist with multidisciplinary team (PCP, dietician, endocrinologist, cardiologist, others)	
Lifestyle intervention[2]	Yes	Yes	Yes
Weight loss recommended if overweight or obese[3]	Yes May benefit from structured weight loss programs, anti-obesity medications, bariatric surgery	Yes Greater need for structured weight loss programs, anti-obesity medications, bariatric surgery	Yes Strong need for structured weight loss programs, anti-obesity medications, bariatric surgery
Pharmacotherapy for NASH	Not recommended	Yes[4,5]	Yes[4,5]
CVD risk reduction[6]	Yes	Yes	Yes
Diabetes care	Standard of care	Prefer medications with efficacy in NASH (pioglitazone, GLP-1 RA)	Prefer medications with efficacy in NASH (pioglitazone, GLP-1 RA)

FIGURE 8.9. Management of NAFLD/NASH.[2]

Case Summary and Closing Points

NAFLD and NASH rates are rising dramatically and serve as the next metabolic pandemic. The number one cause of death in people with NASH is cardiovascular disease. Some emerging tests might be beneficial for staging NASH such as enhanced liver fibrosis test. While there are no FDA-approved treatments for NASH currently, there is much that can be done including targeted screening, noninvasive diagnosis, and treatment based on patient risk with weight loss and cardiovascular risk reduction as foundational therapy.

References

1. Kanwal F, Shubrook JH, Younossi Z, et al. Preparing for the NASH epidemic: a call to action. *Gastroenterology*. 2021;161(3):1030-1042. doi:10.1053/j.gastro.2021.04.074
2. Kanwal F, Shubrook JH, Adams LA. Clinical care pathway for the risk stratification and management of patients with nonalcoholic fatty liver disease. *Gastroenterology*. 2021;161(5):1657-1669. doi:10.1053/j.gastro.2021.07.049
3. Younossi ZM, Felix S, Jeffers T, et al. Performance of the enhanced liver fibrosis test to estimate advanced fibrosis among patients with nonalcoholic fatty liver disease. *JAMA Netw Open*. 2021;4(9):e2123923. doi:10.1001/jamanetworkopen.2021.23923

Index

Note: Page numbers followed by 'f' indicate figures and those followed by 't' indicate tables.